The Developing Child

Recent decades have witnessed unprecedented advances in research on human development. Each book in The Developing Child series reflects the importance of this research as a resource for enhancing children's well-being. It is the purpose of the series to make this resource available to that increasingly large number of people who are responsible for raising a new generation. We hope that these books will provide rich and useful information for parents, educators, child-care professionals, students of developmental psychology, and all others concerned with childhood.

Jerome Bruner, University of Oxford
Michael Cole, Rockefeller University
Barbara Lloyd, University of Sussex
Series Editors

Distress and Comfort

Judy Dunn

Harvard University Press
Cambridge, Massachusetts
1977

Library of Congress Cataloging in Publication Data
Dunn, Judy, 1939-
  Distress and comfort.
  (The Developing child)
  Bibliography: p.
  Includes index.
  1. Infant psychology. I. Title. II. Series.
BF723.I6D86   155.4'22   76-30319
ISBN 0-674-21284-3 (cloth)
ISBN 0-674-21285-1 (paper)

Contents

1	Changing Causes of Distress	1
2	The Newborn Baby	5
3	Why Is the Baby Crying?	17
4	Changes over the Early Months	27
5	Child and Parent in the Early Months	47
6	Crying, Comfort, and Attachments	63
7	The Response to Longer Separations	73
8	Other Cultures	87
9	The Development of Understanding	95
10	So What?	109

References	115
Suggested Reading	121
Index	123

Credits

viii Sam Sweezy (Stock/Boston)

4 George Malave (Stock/Boston)

7 From Peter Wolff, "The Natural History of Crying and Other Vocalisations in Early Infancy." In B. M. Foss, ed., *Determinants of Infant Behavior IV* (London: Methuen, 1969).

10 From J. F. Bernal, "Crying During the First Ten Days of Life and Maternal Responses," *Developmental Medicine and Child Neurology*, 1972, *14*.

16 Julie O'Neil (Stock/Boston)

26 Anna Kaufman Moon (Stock/Boston)

46 Anna Kaufman Moon (Stock/Boston)

52 From L. W. Sander, "Comments on Regulation and Organization in the Early Infant-Caretaker System." In R.J. Robinson, ed., *Brain and Early Behavior* (New York: Academic Press, 1969).

56 Drawing by Sarah Landry. Adapted from I. C. Kaufman and L. A. Rosenblum, "The Reaction to Separation in Infant Monkeys: Anaclitic Depression and Conservation-Withdrawal," *Psychosomatic Medicine*, 1967, *29*.

62 Patricia Hollander Gross (Stock/Boston)

72 Mike Mazzaschi (Stock/Boston)

86 Lorna Marshall (private collection)

94 Anna Kaufman Moon (Stock/Boston)

108 Julie O'Neil (Stock/Boston)

The
Developing
Child

Distress and Comfort

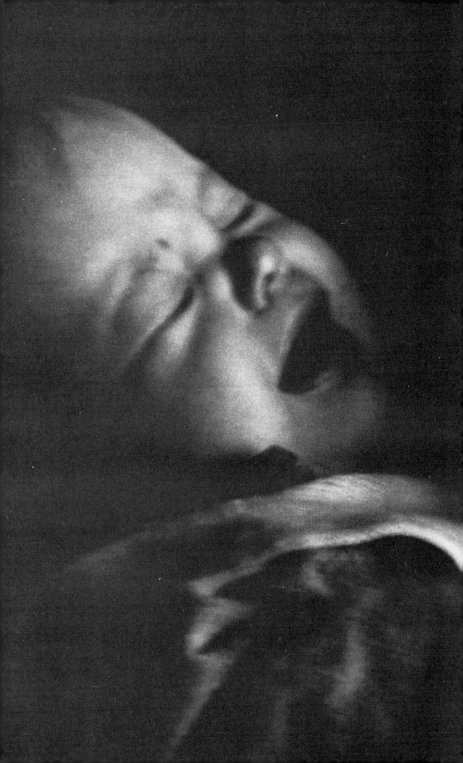

1 / The Changing Causes of Distress

Why a book on distress and comfort in babies? For parents and those caring for young children, great concern centers on the baby's distress. Why is the baby crying—what does the crying mean? Is she hungry when she cries? Will it matter if she's picked up each time she cries? Why does she seem so inconsolable in the evenings? What about comforters—thumbsucking, pacifiers, blankets—will they go on forever if we let her console herself this way? Why are some babies so easy and placid, others so fretful? Will a baby who is irritable and tense grow up to be a difficult child? Why do some babies begin to be shy of unfamiliar people? Why do some cling to their mothers, and others enjoy the attention of strangers? How much do babies miss their mothers if they go out to work, and will distressful separations early on mean that the child is harmed in some long-lasting way? Can we "reverse" the effects of early unhappiness? Does the experience of a loving or an indifferent mother affect the way a baby's confidence and skills of communication develop? How does a baby's intellectual development relate to his early experiences with his parents?

These are questions that matter very much to parents, and in this book we look carefully at what is and what is not known about these issues. But when we examine the results of research in this way, we don't simply gain some useful practical lessons (and a healthy skepticism about much advice that is given to parents). Beyond these urgent practical questions, we also begin to see that what upsets babies and that what provides comfort for them *changes* as they develop. Our spotlight on distress and comfort shows us, quite dramatically, how the baby begins to

1

understand his world, how he responds to it, and how he develops his relationships with people.

Compare the distress of a two-week-old baby, crying vigorously while his mother struggles to bathe him, dry him, dress him, and get his milk ready, with a one-year-old's unhappiness when his mother leaves him and his joy when she returns. It is clear that in this first year the changes in what distresses the baby and what gives comfort reflect great changes in his understanding. The one-year-old's comfort and joy is bound up with his parent, a particular person, and the stage when a baby begins to be comforted by the presence of a particular person marks a profound change in the way he perceives the world. If we think about the situations that upset a child of eighteen months, we can distinguish three different sorts of distress. First, the baby can show distress at a physical situation: he cries when he is cold or has an earache. Second, he can show distress when he recognizes a situation as threatening or wrong in some way: he cries when his favorite car is taken by a bigger child or when his mother leaves him in an unfamiliar house. Third, he can use crying deliberately to get his mother's attention—as a means of achieving an end. In a similar way, comfort can be differentiated: comfort of a "physiological" kind, where warmth is provided for a baby crying when cold and milk for a baby crying when hungry, and "psychological" comfort, which comes from the child's interpretation and understanding of the situation— the comfort provided by the special person whose absence was a cause of distress, and the comfort provided by a familiar person in a strange place.

To make this sort of distinction does not mean that we can necessarily recognize what is distressing a baby on any particular occasion. If something *stops* a baby crying (milk or mother's return), the lack of milk or mother may not have originally caused the crying. There are a number of comforting actions that soothe babies, who can be upset for a wide variety of reasons. But the distinction does highlight the interesting question underlying the changes in what causes distress over the first year. How are these changes related to the baby's developing understanding and to the nature of his relationships with the other people in his world? In the first part of this book, we will be looking to see how changes in crying patterns help us to understand the child's development.

In the second half of the book we turn to the roles that comfort and distress play in the growth of the young child's relationships. How does the way a mother responds to her baby's distress affect the way he behaves and the way he grows up? Does her response to his crying and her way of comforting him influence the growth of a bond between them? We are looking here beyond the issues of "spoiling" to the central question of how a child's early experiences with those who care for him affect his later development. What are the effects on children of being brought up in group care, in extended families, or in institutions? We shall discuss the ideas behind the different views held by psychologists who study social development and compare them with the results of research. The initial focus on distress and comfort then leads us on to a broad range of further questions: the origins of temperamental differences between children, and the effects of these differences on their parents; the importance of the early exchange between parent and baby for the child's developing skills; the beginnings of intentional behavior; the differences between different cultural groups in childrearing. Another question that will recur is the issue of the "biological" importance of crying and comforting: a baby's crying has a very dramatic effect on other people, and we can see how useful this powerful signal system must have been as man evolved. It ensured protection for the young during the long and vulnerable period of infancy. For millions of years babies have been carried or held for most of their early life, provided with constant comfort. What are the consequences today for the baby who is left to "cry it out"? Throughout the book, then, we will keep an eye on the practical implications of the ideas and research for all those concerned with the care of children.

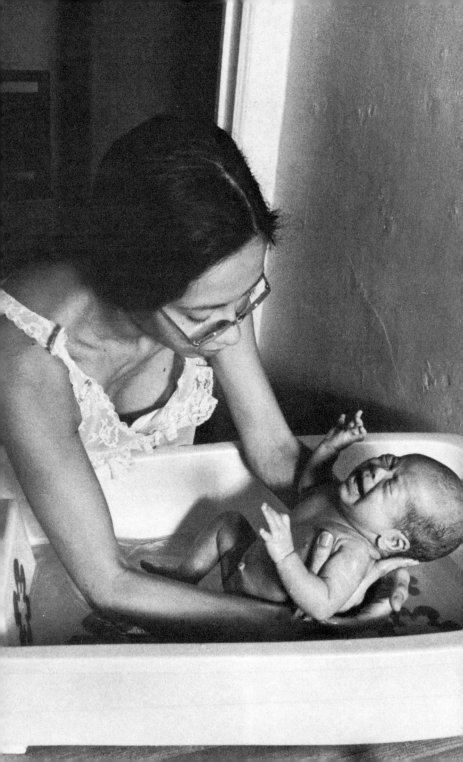

2 / The Newborn Baby

The newborn baby seems helpless, defenseless, and vulnerable. And yet in his crying he possesses a signaling system of enormous strength, through which he exerts an immediate effect on the people around him. Older children, as we all know, use this system of signaling in a highly self-conscious manner to produce effects that seem clearly conceived and deliberately intended. For newborns, crying is plainly not a form of elaborately planned action. Still it can and will be interpreted by adults as a system of intentional communication. But what sort of signaling system is it, and is the message clear for all to read? Are there different natural signals in the system from the moment of birth, or is newborn crying a random expression of distress?

One way to investigate this is to tape-record babies crying in different situations, where we might expect different signals to occur, and to see whether people do hear differences in the crying. Still more fundamentally, we can try to determine whether the crying in each of these different situations has a characteristic sound that adults can identify. In 1968, John Lind, Olé Wasz-Hoeckert, and their colleagues investigated these questions.[1] The problem with their approach was that they had to make *assumptions* about why the baby was crying when they were choosing types of crying to compare. This meant that they had to investigate situations that differed in very crude ways. They looked at (a) the first cry given at delivery—the birth cry; (b) the cry given when the baby was pricked or pinched sharply—the pain cry; (c) the crying of a newborn baby who had not been fed for four hours—the hunger cry.

When tape recordings of these three cry types were played to listeners, they were identified with great accuracy, most of all by midwives, children's nurses, and mothers. The acoustic properties of the cry types can be investigated by a technique called spectrographic analysis. This technique produces a picture (a spectrogram) of the way in which the energy in a child's cry is distributed across the frequency range. Spectrograms of the cry types were analyzed, and particular features of sound were screened out as the best predictors of cry type. On the basis of these features most cry signals recorded in the three situations can be identified at a glance.

But it would be misleading to suggest from this work that babies are born with a number of clearly defined signal cries which a caregiver should be able to recognize and interpret. To begin with, although the third type of cry was called a hunger cry, we do not have evidence of a *causal* relation between hunger and this particular pattern of crying. Moreover, in 1969, Peter Wolff showed that the hunger cry was a basic pattern of rhythmic crying to which infants sooner or later revert—from other types of crying.[2] Even the pain crying produced by a pin prick reverted after some minutes to this pattern (see Figure 1). However, Wolff did find that parents could identify some variations in this basic cry—such as a "mad" cry, when the baby seemed exasperated, a variation of the pain cry, produced by teasing the baby with a pacifier. But he stressed that even on a single day any baby could produce many forms of crying which did not fit into a simple classification of cause and effect. What this suggests is that, although newborn cries given in some extreme situations (birth, pin prick, and so on) can be differentiated and recognized by parents, the everyday crying of a newborn heard by a mother (which in the United States and Europe is often several minutes after the baby has started, since he may be in another room) is not a clearly marked signal of a particular cause of unhappiness. So parents have to decide why a baby is crying on the basis of other information.

First, though, I should note that the detailed and precise analysis of cries made possible with spectrographic techniques has provided doctors with a useful tool for diagnosing abnormalities of the nervous system. In several conditions, the cry is abnormal —for instance, in children with Down's syndrome (mongolism). Doctors studying children whose brains have been injured about the time of birth have found that, while the crying did not

BASIC CRIES

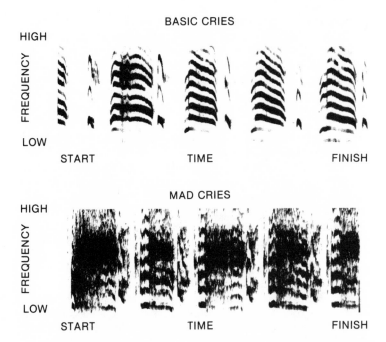

1. *Two spectrograms of a baby crying for about five seconds. These "sound pictures" are constructed so that the louder the sound the darker the mark on the paper. The top picture represents a sequence of four repeated cries by a four-day-old baby boy. The bottom picture shows a sequence of five angry cries by a four-day-old baby girl. The fuzziness in the picture of the mad cries represents the hissing sounds caused by the excess air which the angry baby is forcing through her vocal chords.*

always *sound* different, the spectrographic analysis did enable them to identify relatively clear differences. Spectrographic techniques may well prove useful in finding out the extent of damage to the nervous system that newborns have suffered in the period around birth.

HOW DO PARENTS IDENTIFY CRIES?

In the weeks following the birth, most mothers become increasingly able to distinguish the baby's different forms of crying and vocalizing, and the babies for their part become increasingly able to anticipate their mother's responses. But in the first few weeks the questions of why the baby is crying and what will comfort him are problems that loom very large. What sorts of interpretations do mothers give to the crying they hear at home? There is a great difference from the situation in the cry-type study where the listener was simply told that each cry was either a pain cry, a birth cry, or a hunger cry. At home the choice of possibilities is much wider. Is he hungry, or has he a stomach-ache or gas? Is he bored, angry, overtired? Is he lonely, or just generally miserable? While newborn crying works very well as a way of getting mother's attention, for most mothers in the Western world it hardly amounts to a communication system of great subtlety.

In a study in Cambridge, England, Martin Richards and I found that mothers varied greatly in how they interpreted their babies' crying.[3] In the first place, many were at a loss to explain it, particularly in the case of persistent crying in the evenings. In the second place, most breastfeeding mothers tended to assume that the crying showed that the baby was hungry. Although a few mothers responded by feeding the baby regardless of how long it had been since he was last fed, many breastfeeding mothers felt that if adequately fed he should be happy for three to four hours, and hence that this more frequent crying must be a sign that their milk supply was inadequate. This "inadequacy" was the most common reason for giving up breastfeeding. But in fact the babies of the successful breastfeeders, who continued to feed for over six months, cried just as frequently in the early weeks as did the babies of those mothers who gave up: it seems that it is a general feature of the early stages of breastfeeding for babies to sleep for short periods and to take frequent feeds. We found that mothers who were willing to feed their newborn babies when they cried were more likely to be successful breast-feeders later. This fits with the results of experimental studies comparing breastfeeding success of mothers who feed on demand and those who feed on a stricter four-hour schedule. The mothers in our study who changed over to bottle feeding reported without exception that the baby now cried much less, and they felt that their previous interpretation of his crying had therefore been correct.

Many other reasons were put forward to explain crying in the early weeks besides the hunger interpretation. For crying after a feed, the most common reason given was gas. Many mothers would hold and rub their babies for up to twenty minutes after a feed, often with no burp to show for all this effort at the end. But mothers also attributed crying to psychological causes, particularly by eight weeks or so, and here we found quite marked differences between middle- and working-class mothers. A few mothers attributed crying to boredom—"he gets fed up when on his own"—but these were all middle-class mothers. Others by eight weeks felt that much crying was temper, naughtiness, or crankiness.

But what must be stressed about these parental interpretations of very early crying is that the mothers did not base their interpretation on objective differences in the sound of the crying itself. They relied far more, both for interpretations and for decisions about how to respond, on a whole host of other features, such as how long it was since the baby had last been fed, how well he had fed last time, how peaceful he had been for the last half hour or so, how predictable his sleep-wake pattern usually was, how easy he was to soothe, and so on. Dominating the mother's response—what she decided to do about the crying—was her attitude to spoiling, an issue we will discuss in full below. The importance of these external features in influencing the mothers' decisions about how to respond to crying is illustrated by some results from our Cambridge study. The probability that crying will lead to a mother's feeding the baby is importantly influenced by how much time has passed since the previous feed. It is interesting that mothers of second babies are much more likely to feed a crying baby any time after one and a half hours since the previous feed. The mothers of first babies in our sample, on the other hand, tended to stick more closely to the advice they were given about feeding schedules. In consequence their babies cried a great deal more (Figure 2).

INDIVIDUAL DIFFERENCES IN NEWBORNS' IRRITABILITY

Many mothers who have more than one child will graphically describe how one of their children was always miserable as a tiny baby, grizzling and crying, while another was a placid little angel. Wide differences are indeed reported in every study of

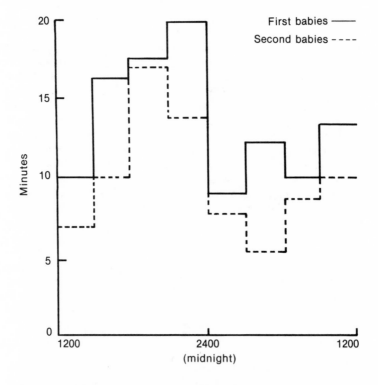

2. *Twenty-four-hour pattern of crying for breastfed babies.*

crying in individual babies during the first two weeks and later. We know, too, that newborn babies differ in how sensitive they are to stimulation, and this means of course that the same sort of maternal caregiving may be experienced very differently by different babies. How much are these differences due to individual characteristics of the baby from birth, and how much are they attributable to his experiences over the first week or so? If they are present at birth, are they related to the sort of labor and delivery mother and baby have gone through? Can we find factors during the pregnancy itself that can be linked to irritability in the period just after birth? As we will see when we look at the interaction between babies and their different caregivers, the way babies behave is affected by the care they have experienced from the earliest days. This means that, even in the first week or so, it is impossible to say definitely that the amount of crying a baby does is either independent of or caused by the sort of care he has received. If we compare the individual crying scores of the babies in our Cambridge study we find that they range in the first week from 10 minutes a day to 190 minutes a day, but we cannot treat these figures as reflections of temperamental differences between the babies, because they may well be dependent on the care and attention the babies have received. However, in an elegant study by Louis Sander, which I discuss in detail in Chapter Four, the effects of differences in caregiving technique were controlled by examining the behavior of different babies with the same foster mother.[4] In this study Sander found that the babies varied greatly in whether they cried at particular points in the sleep-wake cycle: some babies cried in a particular state of drowsiness, others consistently cried at the point of waking. Sander found that there were wide individual differences between babies in the total amount of crying, *even though the babies were looked after by the same nurse in the same situation.* There was also variation in the way crying changed over the first month: in one baby, the changes would be very rapid; in another they would be much slower.

The effects of medication, labor, and delivery. One of our difficulties in describing differences between newborn babies accurately is that in the first few days after birth the baby must adjust to an enormous change in his environment, and must recover from what was often a long-drawn-out delivery. This means that his behavior may vary greatly from day to day; and if we are comparing individual differences between babies it is important to know how stable these differences will be beyond this newborn period. Quite recently T. Berry Brazelton developed a promising new system for looking at differences between newborns. [5] Although most of the reflexes and reactions of newborn babies are studied to pick out abnormalities of the nervous system, Brazelton's system looks particularly at those of the infant's capabilities which are most important to his developing social relationships: for example, how easy it is to console the baby, how quickly he reacts to various sorts of stimulation, and how quickly he calms down on his own. This examination in fact focuses on one of the most interesting features of newborn behavior—the baby's considerable powers of regulating his own state of alertness.

Using Brazelton's system of studying babies, Francis Horowitz and some colleagues found that the babies of mothers who had general anesthesia during delivery were different not only in the immediate postnatal period but at one month after birth. The babies took longer to calm down after being distressed, were less cuddly, and more easily startled. These detailed results parallel other findings indicating that the babies of mothers who have received much medication may be more irritable. In our Cambridge study we found that babies who had been born after a longer labor or with more drugs were more likely to cry frequently and sleep in short bouts during the newborn period. Of course, when we find a link between difficult delivery and early irritability in the baby, or between prenatal maternal anxiety and newborn irritability, we cannot necessarily pinpoint the cause of the link. For instance, differences between the fetuses could *contribute* to a difficult labor—and quite separately to individual differences in the amount of crying the babies did; the labor itself is not necessarily the factor.

Another possibility is that the mother's anxiety, leading to the longer labor, might also independently cause irritability in the baby in the period following birth. Several studies have found that mothers rated as highly anxious during pregnancy had babies who were more irritable or difficult. We don't know much about the physiological effects of anxiety in pregnancy on the baby before birth. Of course, if the description and observation of the babies were made several months after birth, it could well be that the effect was in part a postnatal one: perhaps the mothers who were rated as anxious during pregnancy were still behaving anxiously in the weeks after the birth. However, at least two studies have found that the newborn babies of anxious mothers were more irritable. Even so, it is hard to discern whether the link is a direct prenatal one, or whether it is that more anxious mothers have more difficult labors and that these lead to the differences between babies. There is an intricate tangle of possible causes, and to sort it out we need information on the causes of the anxiety, the physiological effects associated with the anxiety, the course of labor and delivery, and the state and behavior of the baby when he arrives.

Although people have tried to assess the effects of delivery or of maternal prenatal anxiety by using "crying scores," these do not on their own tell us much about, say, a baby's temperament. Many other factors have to be taken into account as well. We have good reason to expect, for example, that, for a mother-baby pair who have experienced a long labor and a high level of maternal medication, feedings may go much less smoothly than for a mother-baby pair who have had a shorter drug-free labor. If a feed has not been very successful, it is very likely that the baby will sleep for a shorter period and cry earlier than if the feed had been satisfactory. The irritability may then be a reflection of the feeding pattern rather than a direct consequence of the effects of the delivery and drugs on the baby's nervous system. In our Cambridge study we found that babies who had experienced a long labor were more likely to have feeding difficulties, as well as to cry frequently and have shorter sleeps.

Sex differences.   Reports on differences between the behavior of newborn boys and of newborn girls do not all tell the same story. Most of the differences that have been confirmed, such as differences in sensitivity and in discrimination of taste, do not bear directly on the issue of comfort and distress. But the boy babies in one study by Howard Moss were more irritable by the age of three weeks than the girls.[6] This finding raises two points of interest. First, it is well established that male babies are more vulnerable to stress at the time of birth. This means that in any sample of babies that is not carefully screened for birth problems, there will be more boys whose behavior is affected by a difficult delivery. It is possible that for this reason they will be more irritable, unpredictable, or difficult. The second point concerns the effects of circumcision. Studies have shown that the operation may have immediate effects on the baby's level of excitability and his sleeping and crying behavior. The operation may be followed by prolonged wakefulness and fussing and crying. There is a real possibility that some of the reported newborn sex differences, notably absent in Europe where circumcision is rare, are in fact differences in behavior arising from the operation. Some studies have shown, for instance, that the behavior of uncircumcised boys is no different from that of girls, whereas circumcised boys do show considerable differences.

Cross-cultural studies. Several comparative studies have looked at newborn babies of different cultures. When the Freedmans compared Chinese-American and European-American babies, the Chinese-American babies were found to be much calmer, more passive in response to unpleasant stimulation.[7] Although there were no differences in the amount of crying during the test, the Chinese babies were much easier to soothe, and stopped crying as soon as they were picked up and spoken to. They were also better at self-quieting.

Another study by Berry Brazelton compared a group of Zinacanteco Indian babies from Mexico with babies from the United States; all the babies had had drug-free deliveries. The Indian babies stayed in a quiet alert state for longer periods of time than the American babies, and the American babies cried more intensely and slept more deeply. In yet another study, Uruguayan babies were found to be easier to soothe than American babies. These differences between cultures are discussed in more detail in Chapter Eight.

We are a long way from understanding how far the differences in newborn irritability reviewed in this chapter reflect differences in the experience of the babies before birth, or genetic differences, or differences stemming from labor and delivery procedures, or differences in the experience of the babies after birth. What we do know is that, whatever their origins, they have important consequences for the interaction between babies and their parents or caregivers. We turn next to the question that puzzles so many parents—why is the baby crying?

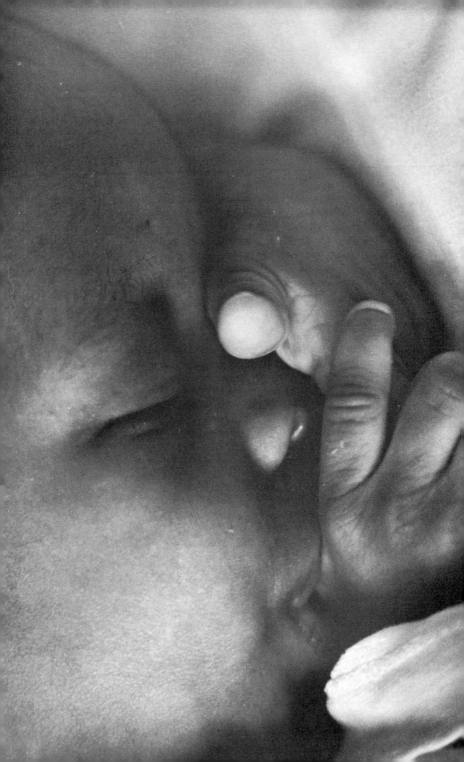

3 / Why Is the Baby Crying?

If you watch a newborn baby for several hours, you will notice that he goes through different states of wakefulness, restlessness, and sleepiness. Sometimes he'll be sleeping deeply, with regular breathing, no small movements; sometimes although his eyes are closed he breathes much more irregularly, twitches and stirs in his sleep; sometimes he lies awake, calm and alert; sometimes he actively moves arms, legs, and body around; sometimes he is restless and fussing, sometimes crying vigorously. How are these states related? Is there a simple continuum of restlessness with deep sleep at one end and crying at the other? What sort of reaction from his mother will make the baby more likely to shift from crying to calm or sleep, and do these reactions help us understand the relationship between the various states?

STATES OF CONSCIOUSNESS

These questions are important to us in our attempts to understand what distresses and what comforts a very young baby, because the same noise or movement will make a baby cry when he is in one state of wakefulness or sleepiness but not when he is in another. But there are two ways of describing these different states of alertness, ways we ought to be careful to distinguish. One way is simply to describe the baby's behavior; here we can distinguish a number of different states, depending on the criteria we choose. The most usual way of categorizing the baby's state is based on whether his eyes are open or closed, how regular his breathing is, and whether he is actively moving around or crying. Using these criteria five different states can be distinguished: (1) deep sleep, (2) light sleep, when the baby has his eyes

17

closed but breathes irregularly and shows small movements, (3) quiet alert, when his eyes are open but he is still and attentive, (4) active awake, when he moves vigorously, and (5) crying. Drowsiness, when the baby breathes irregularly and intermittently opens and closes his eyes, is usually described as a transition state, since careful studies show this state does not usually last more than three minutes at a time.

The way a baby responds to noises and movements depends on which of these states he is in. In deep sleep, he is buffered from mild stimulation—either from the outside world or from his own body, although more extreme noises, abrupt movements, or pains can break into sleep. As time passes, and the period since he was last fed increases, the baby becomes more susceptible to both internal and external stimulation, and is more easily awakened. In lighter sleep, mild stimulation that was not enough to start movements when he was deeply asleep now start him thrashing around. When the baby is in a quiet alert state he will attend to something interesting you give him to look at, and indeed you can keep him in this quiet state for many minutes. Peter Wolff showed that you can bring a drowsy baby repeatedly back to a state of alert inactivity by giving him interesting things to look at.[1] If a baby's attention is caught in this way he will tend to stop thrashing his arms and legs about. But once he is really crying and struggling, only active pacifying techniques or very great fatigue can calm him down.

The other way of describing the baby's different states of alertness is to use terms such as "level of arousal" or "level of consciousness." When this arousal language is used, it is assumed that the various states of alertness are on a continuum of some sort of central nervous excitation. Therefore, a model of this kind would explain the effectiveness of particular comforting techniques by their ability to reduce the baby's arousal level—to move him down on the scale. But careful work on the relationship of the body and the nervous system, for instance by John Hutt, Heinz Prechtl, and their colleagues,[2] has shown that this is not the right way to think of the baby's different states. The language of arousal level is interpretative, and in fact assumes that the central nervous system is organized in a particular way; we now know enough about the brain to see that this assumption is not justified. "Arousal" is a rough and ready notion: the various ways we might measure it, such as heartrate, breathing rate, and blood pressure, do not always increase or decrease together in the different states. When we describe actions that calm a baby and lead to a change in his state, we are very far from being able to explain what is happening in terms of the baby's central nervous system.

But our simple description of the five states classified according to the baby's breathing, movements, and eyes also has limitations. It would not differentiate, for example, the baby who was crying vigorously when he had not been fed for four hours from the baby crying after a prick on his heel or from the baby crying after being teased and frustrated with a pacifier. These babies would respond very differently to different comforting techniques. Another limitation was pointed out by Wolff, who observed that drowsiness while falling asleep was not identical with drowsiness when waking up, even though the baby's appearance might be similar. Wolff stressed that it was important to take account of the steps leading up to a particular state: the baby who is alert after a period of drowsiness may behave rather differently from a baby who is alert after a period of crying.

We do, however, know enough to stress how important it is to take account of a baby's state. How a baby responds to particular stimulation (unless it is extremely unpleasant) *does* depend on his state, and this is particularly true of the way he responds to people. The best possible state for the intimate exchange of gaze between mother and child is one where the baby is calm and alert. Our interest then in the calming effect of a mother's picking up a crying baby is not simply in the part this plays in removing a cause of distress—that in state X he was uncomfortable but in his mother's arms he is in state Y and is comfortable. Notice rather the way the baby stops thrashing, becomes calm and attentive, scans the world and gazes at his mother's face. She returns his intent gaze, smiles, nods, and talks to him. It is when he is in this calm attentive state that he can begin to know his mother's face and voice, can begin to take part in the reciprocal exchanges of looks, sounds, and movements—in the "conversations" that are so important in the development of their relationship.

Watching the shifts in babies' states of consciousness has made us aware of an interesting dimension of a baby's abilities at birth: a baby does have some powers of self-quieting, of controlling his own exposure to the environment and cutting off too much stimulation. But these abilities are, of course, very limited. The infant is frequently overwhelmed by stimuli over which he has absolutely no control; and when he is, the result is distress. Although some of the causes of such distress are fairly obvious, there has in fact been rather little systematic work on the range of causes in the early days. The study of crying by Peter Wolff stands very much alone (in discussing these early sources of distress I have drawn heavily on his work).[3]

CAUSES OF DISTRESS

Hunger. In our Cambridge study we asked the mothers of newborn babies what they thought lay behind their babies' crying during the first weeks. The mothers who were breastfeeding thought that hunger was by far the most common cause. Studies looking at how much babies cry before and after feedings certainly confirm that babies cry much less after feedings, and that this is not simply a response to being held. But feeding involves many different factors, any or all of which might have a soothing effect: sucking, swallowing, having a full stomach, absorbing nourishment. Wolff was able to look separately at the effects of swallowing and sucking, on the one hand, and having a full stomach, on the other, by studying babies who because of medical problems were being fed through tubes to the stomach. He could separate the effects of swallowing from those of sucking by allowing babies to suck at a pacifier while the food went straight to the stomach through the tube, and he could isolate the effects of sucking and swallowing from the effects of having a full stomach. Although these experiments were done on only seven babies, and must therefore be interpreted cautiously, the results consistently showed that a full stomach, rather than sucking or swallowing, seemed to be most effective at stopping the hungry newborn's rhythmic crying.

Temperature. Temperature and humidity both have important effects on the amount of time babies sleep, on their activity and crying. Wolff found that babies kept at 88-90 degrees cried less and slept more than when kept at 78 degrees. Though wet or dirty diapers in themselves are not sufficient to cause crying, if the wet diaper leads to cooling, the drop in temperature is a potent cause of distress. Wolff comments that the cooler temperature itself may not cause crying, but that since babies sleep more deeply when warm, colder babies may be more responsive to stimulation and so more liable to cry for other reasons.

Clothing and contact. Wolff also made some interesting observations on the way babies responded to nakedness and skin contact. Seven out of eighteen newborn babies, from the third day on, began to cry when they were undressed, even when the temperature was controlled and when they had been awake and content immediately before their clothes were taken off. This effect was consistent, and indeed increasingly vigorous, over the second and third weeks. To soothe these babies it was not enough to cover them with a blanket or to cover the arms and legs only. It was swaddling or providing cloth contact for the front of the chest or tummy that worked, and the texture of the cloth was important. Plastic or rubber was less effective than toweling or blanketing. In several cultures babies are provided with constant contact comfort by being swaddled or bound. In other cultures babies are in constant skin contact with their mothers or caregivers, by being carried on their bodies in slings. As we will see later, crying is very unusual in those societies where babies have constant contact.

Pain, colic, and evening crying. While it is clear that a prick on the heel or some other physical assault leads directly to crying, how much of a baby's crying during his normal routine is due to internal pain such as stomachache or gas is not easy to judge.

The disagreements among pediatricians and psychologists about what causes the regular evening crying so common among babies illustrate this difficulty. It is agreed by many doctors that regular crying in the evening is very common among babies who otherwise seem healthy. As the pediatrician Ronald Illingworth comments: "The outstanding impression given by the colicky baby, except in the evening, is that he is a well, happy, thriving, well-fed and well-managed baby with nothing wrong with him."[4]

In our Cambridge study more than half the babies cried regularly in the evenings at two months of age; for many this was just intermittent fussing, which could be soothed by nursing, but for some the distress was extreme. In Illingworth's study, twenty-one out of a hundred healthy babies were considered to suffer from colic. Illingworth carefully investigated the range of causes to which colic has been attributed by various writers: overfeeding, underfeeding, allergy, constipation, diarrhea, too much gas in the bowel, parents picking the baby up too much, parents picking the baby up too little. He found no evidence for any of these causes, and suggested that in the extreme cases the most likely explanation lay in a localized obstruction of the passage of gas in the colon. He stressed that spoiling was unlikely to be the original cause of the regular evening crying, since in his study thirty-three out of forty-nine cases began in the hospital before the baby was at home with the parents.

Illingworth could not suggest any reason why the crying should happen predominantly in the evening. It is often suggested that the "evening peak" is due to the mother's tiredness and busyness in the evening, with the implication that the mother is less attentive to the baby than earlier in the day. But the data from our Cambridge study show that, in this sample at least, the babies were certainly not unattended to in the evening.

The breastfed babies cried more in the evenings than the bottle-fed babies in this study and were more difficult to soothe by holding. These two findings are compatible with the idea that hunger contributes to the evening peak in crying, since the quantity of breast milk is often lower in the late afternoon feeds. But the point remains that several of the bottle-fed babies also showed an evening peak in crying.

Violent or sudden stimulation. Intense or sudden changes in the level of stimulation the baby is receiving by any of the sensory systems—eye, ear, balance—make the baby startle and begin to cry.

SOURCES OF COMFORT

We have seen that in some cases we *can* infer what is causing the distress from the specific action that soothes the baby, as in

Wolff's experiments on feeding or undressing. But more generally there are ways that caregivers all over the world use to soothe and calm babies—rocking, patting, cuddling, swaddling, giving suck on breast or pacifier. Two features of such "everyday" soothing techniques that experimental studies have underlined as important are: (1) the provision of a background of constant or rhythmic rather than variable stimulation; (2) the reduction of the amount of sensation that the baby receives from his *own* movements (called the "proprioceptive feedback"). Swaddling, for example, when properly done provides a baby with constant touch stimulation, and it also reduces the amount of movement the baby can make and thus the amount of stimulation he gets from his own movements.

It is by no means always easy to figure out exactly how the calming technique is working. Sucking on a pacifier, for example, is extremely effective at stopping a baby's crying. Jerome Bruner has shown that sucking relaxes the movements of the gut and of the major muscles, and that it also reduces the number of eye movements the baby makes when given something patterned to look at. While the baby is sucking in this way, not only is the stimulation from his mouth regular and rhythmic, but his random thrashing about is greatly reduced. The causes of this calming down are not quite clear: it could be that the sucking reduces the active thrashing (and with it the feedback of sensation from arms and legs to the brain); or it could be that the effect is in the opposite direction—that the sucking itself calms the baby down and so stills the movements. But, either way, the calming effect of sucking is particularly interesting because it shows us one way in which the baby's actions control his own state even as a newborn.

To study the soothing effect of rocking, Anthony Ambrose developed a rocking "machine" to find out which particular aspects of rocking were most effective. He discovered that when rocked at a rate of 60 rocks per minute, with a swing of 2-3/4 inches, babies invariably stopped crying.[5] We don't yet know what the effects of this rhythmic stimulation are on other aspects of "arousal," such as heart and breathing rates. But a study by Yvonne Brackbill showed that constant stimulation—through sound, light, swaddling, or temperature—increased the amount of time spent quietly asleep and reduced the time the baby spent

crying, his heartrate, breathing rate, and amount of movement.[6]
If two or more of these were combined (swaddling with sound),
the drop in different aspects of arousal increased cumulatively.
Interestingly, Brackbill found that, although the continuous
stimulation did decrease the time the child spent crying, and increased the time he spent asleep, it did not affect the time spent
in other states such as drowsiness or quiet wakefulness. That is,
the sleepiness produced by the continuous stimulation did not
occur at the expense of the time he spent quietly awake.

Brackbill compared the effects of the different kinds of continuous stimulation; she found that, while all four types of continuous stimulation pacified the babies, swaddling was overwhelm-
ingly the most effective.

Thumbsucking. Psychologists do not agree about either the
origins or the consequences of thumbsucking. According to one
view, thumbsucking is a natural exercise by which the baby effectively comforts himself. The origins of the habit have been
linked, very plausibly, with two particular reflexes that can be
elicited in newborn babies.

If you stroke the face of a newborn baby in the area around
his mouth, he will turn his head toward your stroking finger,
opening his mouth. This "searching" for the stimulus is a reflex,
known as the rooting reflex, which can be elicited during the first
three months in babies. It is clearly very useful, as is the "placing" reflex that follows rooting: the baby has searched for the
stimulus with open mouth, fastens onto it, and begins to suck.
The two reflexes together mean that a newborn baby is quite
skillful at finding and fastening onto the nipple when he is held
in his mother's arms. When he goes to sleep in a crib his hands
are close to his face and often touch it. In this situation he is very
likely to root for and find his fingers. Lorna Benjamin found that
if you cover a baby's hands during the three-month period while
the rooting and placing reflexes last, thereby preventing him
from finding his fingers when he is put to sleep, he is much less
likely to develop the habit.[7]

A rather different view of thumbsucking relates the habit
more directly to the feeding pattern that the mother has established. One version of this view suggests that thumbsucking
comes from an unsatisfied need to suck. Thumbsucking reflects a

feeding pattern where the mother has not allowed the baby enough sucking experience; to stop the baby from sucking his thumb, she is advised to increase his feeding time. Directly opposed to this version is the idea that sucking is associated with the baby's pleasure in feeding, which suggests that thumbsucking can be reduced if the feeding time is shortened, with the link between sucking and the pleasure of feeding then weakened. To test these opposing views Lorna Benjamin carried out experiments with rhesus monkeys, allowing them varying amounts of sucking experience. The monkeys with more sucking experience during feeds showed more thumbsucking—which supports the second version.

Once the thumbsucking habit has become established and continues beyond the age of six or seven months, it is very hard to break and may continue till the child is four or five years old. The persistence with which the child clings to the habit is similar to that with which other self-comforting habits are retained.

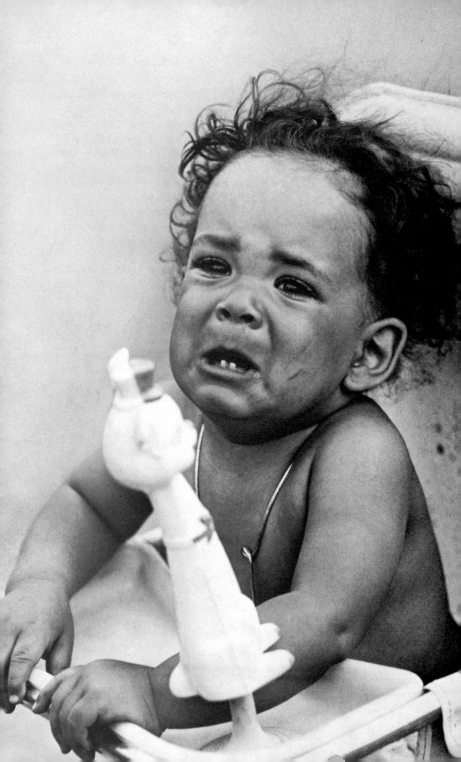

4 / Changes over the Early Months

Although newborn crying still retains its mysteries, most notably colic, much early crying can be directly attributed to immediate changes in the infant's physical state. If the baby becomes hungry, feels pain, or experiences sudden movement, he cries. The adaptive value of such crying is not difficult to understand. Crying provides a signal to the parent that something is wrong and, in its compelling way, prompts the parent to intervene. However, as the infant begins to grow, and his appreciation of the world around him begins to develop, the causes of crying very quickly become more complicated. By examining these complications, we can begin to get some idea of just how fast the infant's understanding of the world around him begins to take shape.

CHANGES IN CAUSES OF CRYING AND IN COMFORTING

Peter Wolff noted that in the first week babies responded by crying when he "teased" them by repeatedly removing a pacifier from their mouths, and that in the second week bottle-fed babies began to cry when their feed was interrupted. In our Cambridge study we found that this would happen by the eighth day after birth. Even as early as this, a baby can be upset by frustrations that are "psychological" rather than simply physiological changes in arousal. With breastfed babies, crying during feeds was much more rare, and Wolff suggested this might be because breastfed babies were given a much longer first round of sucking than bottle-fed babies. This explanation seems very likely: the breastfed babies in our study were allowed to suck for much longer before a round was ended, and there was a striking difference between the breast- and bottle-fed babies in the amount of control that they were given over ending a round of sucking. In the bottle-feeding situation it was the mother who ended 75 percent of the rounds, but the breastfed babies were just as likely as their mothers to end the sucking.

During the next two to three weeks, with the baby's increasing interest in the world around him, and his increasing control over his own attention, it becomes much easier to soothe him by showing him something interesting (though not if he is crying frantically). Already by the second week we find that the human voice is more effective at calming a crying baby than a rattle or bell. His attention and interest are more drawn by human than by nonhuman sounds. Visually, the human face does not seem to be any more effective than an inanimate object until the baby is about a month old. By this time, someone looking and talking to him does sometimes stop the baby's fussing, and he will watch with great interest. Not only this, but he will often cry for a few minutes when the person leaves his presence.

This crying at being left seems to vary greatly between individual babies—some always cry at being left, others only occasionally. But although its incidence varies, it is clear that the change reflects the baby's increasing sociability and his interest in people. If a feed is interrupted at five or six weeks, most babies are so interested in what is going on around them that they don't object at all. Wolff showed that the crying at being left is not yet directed at particular people; if his mother leaves and there is someone else talking to him, he won't cry. It also does not look as if the crying at being left at this stage is *intentional* crying—that is, crying in order to get someone back. The baby cries as soon as he is left and calms down after a minute or so; if the person reappears, and then repeats his departure, the departure again leads to a few minutes of fussing—but the baby is also increasingly proficient at calming himself (by thumbsucking, for instance).

Frustration and teasing. As the baby develops new skills of coordination, and new interests and activities, he can be frustrated in new ways. At two or three months, when he is very interested in handling objects and looking at them, he may cry if something he is holding is removed. Wolff points out that it does not irritate a younger baby if you remove a rattle from his hands and that, again *after* hand-eye coordination is well established, it is less likely to lead to this kind of protest. What frustrates a baby depends on the meaning and interest that objects or actions have for him at his particular stage of development. Once particular objects have a special meaning for him, removal of these of course causes great distress.

CHANGES IN REACTION TO PEOPLE

We have seen that at five or six weeks some babies cry at being left. Now consider these two observations:

> A ten-week-old baby is lying in his crib. His mother, tidying the blankets, leans over him talking and smiling, while the baby coos and "talks" back. The mother leaves the room to greet a visitor. The baby cries. The visitor, who has not seen the baby before, comes over, leans down, smiles, and talks to the baby. The baby stops crying and smiles as the visitor picks him up.

> An eight-month-old baby is playing on her mother's knee, when her mother puts her down and leaves the room to answer the door. As the visitor enters, the baby cries. When the visitor attempts to comfort her by picking her up, the baby cries more frantically until the mother returns and holds her. Then the baby calms down. From her mother's lap she first stares and later smiles at the visitor.

Notice a crucial change between the two situations. The baby at eight months protests at being left, as does the ten-week-old, but it is now her *mother's* departure she minds. The visitor, far from comforting her, seems to upset her more. She no longer treats people as interchangeable companions; separation from her mother has taken on a new meaning.

Now we know that babies are able to discriminate their mothers, or familiar caregivers, from other people very early on in the first year. Wolff found, for example, that by the fifth week of life the mother's voice was more effective than the observer's at producing sound from the baby. Leon Yarrow found that by one month 38 percent of them were showing positive reactions to the mother but not toward a stranger.

The distress shown by the eight-month-old in the second situation therefore does not mean that she has *just* learned to distinguish her mother from others. What it does mean is that she is missing her mother in a different way, and that she now remembers her when she is absent. The change then reflects something very profound in the way her memory is working and in her ability to picture to herself people who are absent. There is a lot of evidence to suggest that there are indeed fundamental changes going on in babies' powers of recall during the second half of the first year. Since Jean Piaget drew attention to the gradual development of children's understanding that an object continues to exist even when the child cannot see it, there have been many studies that have examined the growth of this understanding. This capacity is not only of profound importance to the child's understanding about the objects in his world, but it also changes enormously the way he relates to his family and friends. It means that not only does he recognize his mother when she is there, but also that it is no longer true that she is "out of sight, out of mind": he will miss her when she is gone. His tie with those he loves can now span space and time. Perhaps the most striking aspects of this new dimension to his relationships are, on the one hand, his anxiety and distress when left by those he loves and, on the other, the way in which their presense transforms his behavior. In the second of the cases described above, the baby eventually enjoyed the stranger's presence from the safety of her mother's lap. Before looking in detail at the part comfort and distress play in the child's social relationships, there is another aspect of his new and specific responses to people which must be examined, his changing reactions to strangers.

CHANGING REACTIONS TO STRANGERS

Gordon Bronson observed repeatedly the reactions of a group of thirty-two babies to the approach of a strange person over the age period of three to nine months.[1] With some of the three-month-olds, Bronson noted a pattern of wariness in the reaction to the stranger: "Typically, after greeting the stranger with a passing smile the infant would stare intently for some 15-30 seonds, then begin to frown, breathe heavily, and finally start to cry." The pattern was unpredictable, but was characterized by the long stare before the baby began to cry. By six months about half the children were consistently upset by the stranger's presence, though how they reacted was strongly influenced by whether they were in their mother's arms or apart from her. They rarely cried if they were held by the mother and in fact usually smiled. When on their own, or held by the stranger, many did cry. Why were the babies afraid?

The observation that new or unfamiliar sights make animals and people alert, attentive, and possibly also fearful has been investigated in many ways. Recent studies have shown that from very early on babies can be upset when someone they are familiar with behaves oddly. Experiments by Genevieve Carpenter in which a baby saw his mother's face looking at him, intent, unsmiling, and motionless—not her usual animated conversational self—produced much distress. Donald Hebb thirty years ago pointed out that, with animals, fear was evoked by events that were different or *discrepant* from previous experience. From this idea a general theory was developed about the relation between an unfamiliar event and the reaction to it. Central to this "discrepancy hypothesis" is the idea that the amount of attention an animal pays to an event is determined by how different that event is from mental "representation" or stored memory of similar events. The theory tries to explain why the animal may show fear in some unfamiliar situations (rather than simply becoming alert) by suggesting that whether the animal approaches, or is fearful and avoids, depends on how the event differs from the representation in the animal's mind. If the event is very similar to this mental representation or "schema," the animal is bored and no longer attends; if the event is moderately different, the animal is interested (and may, if human, feel pleasure); if the event is very different, the animal cannot assimilate the event to its mental representation. The result of this too-great discrepancy is that the animal becomes distressed and avoids the novel situation.

According to this theory, then, our eight-month-old's fearful reaction to the stranger picking her up and the reaction of the six-month-olds in Bronson's study were both provoked by the "mismatch" between the stranger's face and the babies' remembered images of the people they saw regularly. Although there are many problems involved in this sort of explanation, it is a useful way in which to start thinking about what these changes in the baby's reactions might signify. The explanation depends on the assumption that the child possesses a central pattern formed from the characteristics of the faces he knows, and that when he looks at the stranger he recalls these patterns in order to make the comparison. Not only does he "know" his mother now, but he uses this knowledge in order to judge whether other people are unfamiliar. The idea of a central but recallable inner picture of the mother helped to explain the change in babies' responses to their mother's absence in the second half of the first year. So far so good. But how well does the discrepancy idea account for the baby's unease or wariness of the stranger? For some observations the story fits very well. For example, according to the discrepancy theory wariness reactions should, when they first appear, be uncertain and should appear only after the infant has examined the stranger's face at length. This is exactly what Bronson found. He also suggested that we would expect infants to become more wary as they became more certain in their discrimination of strangers. This he indeed found between four and six and a half months. However, there is no independent evidence to show whether babies' abilities to perceive improve generally in this period; so in itself this observation does not help us to assess the discrepancy idea.

Bronson suggested that part of the explanation for why new objects were less frightening than new people was that the objects were rarely a variant of a familiar object. He put forward an interesting version of the standard discrepancy theory. We know that by the third month of life babies are delighted by events that follow from their own acts (this is well shown by some of the research on smiling, for instance), and are upset if their own behavior with other people fails to produce the reaction they expect. Bronson suggested that, as the baby begins to be more aware of the predictability of social encounters, he may be made wary by behavior that "doesn't fit" with his own behavior. In the study the stranger's behavior was persistent and was not sensitive to the baby's reaction (that is, he didn't go away). So Bronson argued then that wariness depends not only on the perception of discrepancy between the stimulus situation and the baby's inner representations, but also on whether the baby finds the person's *behavior* predictable, related to his own behavior.

Difficulties with the discrepancy theory.   There are, however, some very serious difficulties with trying to understand all incidents of fearful behavior in young children in terms of the discrepancy idea. It seems more reasonable to take the view that some but not all fearfulness is caused by discrepancy between a child's familiar experiences and an unusual event. For example, it is clear that in many real-life incidents where young children are frightened, it is the association with earlier unpleasant experiences—not the discrepancy itself—that leads to distress.

There are in fact two major problems in using the discrepancy idea. First, how do we decide what is *more* or *less* discrepant? Our only measure can be the child's reaction, since we cannot know what internal pattern he will be comparing the event with. As we will see, there is good evidence to suppose that the baby is not operating simply on an assessment of "how much like mother is this?" Second, it is a striking fact that many of the situations that are most potent in upsetting babies—loud noises, strange sights, tossing the baby about—are exactly the situations that produce delighted laughter in slightly different contexts! One study by Alan Sroufe and his colleagues found that the sight of mother wearing a mask produced pleasure and laughter in the great majority of babies when it happened at home. But it led to distress and crying in the laboratory.[2] The simple discrepancy between mother's face and mother-wearing-mask cannot account for why the babies were happy in one situation and frightened in the other. Discrepancy certainly seems to be important in leading to excitement, but whether the excitement leads to pleasure or to fear seems to depend on a complex of other factors, such as where the baby is, whom he is with, how tired or cheerful he is feeling, and so on.

Take, for instance, Sroufe's observation of a mother of a fifteen-month-old, who by picking the baby up by the heels produced squeals of laughter. Moments later the baby became upset as a stranger came in. When, after calming him, the mother again picked the baby up the her heels, the baby cried. It is difficult to see how the discrepancy idea can explain how the same event can produce both laughter and tears in the same baby within such a short time. And the same objection applies to another version of the theory, developed by Jerome Kagan, which holds that whether fear or laughter is produced in an aroused baby is determined by how easily the baby manages to match or assimilate what he sees with his inner representation.[3]

Sroufe suggests that one way of explaining the differences in the child's response in different contexts is to think of the child's considering and "evaluating" the situation. According to this idea, the baby brings to any situation a particular threshold for reacting to new events, a predisposition to react with pleasure or fear. This predisposition is influenced by the baby's temperament, his state of alertness, where he is, whom he is with, what has been happening, his relation with his parents, and so forth. When he becomes alert to the strange person or situation, this predisposition will determine how he evaluates the situation. Evaluation is of course a very vague term—it stresses the thinking involved in assessing the situation. The baby is seen as "judging" whether a new stimulus is threatening. This stress on the thinking involved seems justified by two different sorts of evidence.

The evidence that there are marked age changes in the way babies react to strange situations suggests that what underlies the way older infants respond is an increasing intellectual sophistication. The six-month-old babies in Sroufe's study were not affected by differences in context—by familiarity with the situation and such—in the way the ten-month-olds were. Recall the evidence already discussed on the changes in the baby's reaction to his mother's absence—and the mental processes underlying this. Changes in the source of distress depend greatly on changes in intellectual functioning.

Detailed observation of the behavior of the babies when they saw their mothers put on a mask fits with the idea that a baby evaluates events. All the babies froze, stared at the mask, and their heartrates decelerated. At this stage there were no signs of pleasure or fear. Some of the babies then began to look fearful, their heartrates increased again, and crying began. With others, the heartrate decelerated further, and they began to smile and laugh.

More doubts about whether the discrepancy theory is really useful as an explanation of why children react with fear sometimes and with pleasure at other times were raised by the intriguing observations of Michael Lewis and Jeanne Brooks.[4] Most mothers have noticed that their babies are very much interested in other children. Lewis and Brooks systematically examined how young babies reacted to the approach of strange children as well as strange adults, and they found that they reacted positively to child strangers. They also examined how the baby reacted when, by the use of mirrors, it appeared that the baby was being approached by himself. This time the babies reacted with as much delight as they did to the approach of their mothers. This is very difficult to explain if, as has been supposed, the child makes judgments about familiarity and incongruity using the mother as reference point. The child stranger would be more different from the mother than a female adult stranger, and yet the children showed fear at the approach of the female adult stranger. Lewis suggests that these results imply that the baby does not only compare strange faces with his mother's, but also with *his own*. In some sense, then, the child stranger is recognized by the baby as like himself and therefore not threatening. The differentiation between self and others must be taking place at the time when the child is differentiating mother from others. Do we have to assume, then, that all children have seen reflections of themselves? This seems unlikely. But the idea that the child will have several familiar reference points with which to compare new people certainly makes good sense.

Such research is beginning to outline the way in which the baby begins to categorize "self." It looks as if between nine and eighteen months, for instance, the baby begins to have some sense of the category of gender. Lewis found that girl babies were more frightened of male adult strangers than boy babies were; and that babies between nine and eighteen months preferred looking at pictures of babies of the same sex as themselves.

THE NATURE OF WARINESS, FEAR, OR DISTRESS

We are still a very long way from knowing how to explain why some situations are frightening to a baby and others exciting and pleasurable. Up to now I have used terms like "wariness" and "fear" quite casually. Do we have any grounds for distinguishing the feelings that babies have in different situations or at different ages? It certainly seems justified to talk about fear of strangers when a ten-month-old shrinks away, screams, and clings to his mother as a new adult tries to pick him up. How about a younger child? There are a number of issues we should examine.

What is the baby feeling? How we label behavior does tend to prejudge its emotional meaning: if we label alert and attentive behavior as "wariness," it suggests a negative quality, perhaps unnecessarily. What about using measures of physiological changes in the body to distinguish different emotional states? When animals or people are frightened, or concentrating on something, there are marked changes in the rate at which the heart beats and in the way the blood supply is distributed to other parts of the body. When we are frightened, our heartrate and the blood supply to our muscles increase, to prepare us for "fight or flight." There is much of interest now in the use of physiological measurements such as heartrate to describe the emotional reactions of children. Sroufe has shown that, if we know the changes in heartrate when a baby faces a new situation, we can predict how the baby's facial expression and gaze behavior will change. However, we have to remember that there is in general no simple relationship between the feelings people report, the behavior and expressions they show, and the details of their physiological changes; so taking physiological measures may get us no closer to what the baby is feeling than watching his behavior will.

Changes in the nature of wariness. A number of the mothers in Gordon Bronson's sample reported that at around nine months their babies developed a specific fear or dislike for a particular person. The reaction was always immediate and consistent, and it seems fair enough to suppose that it was because the babies remembered these particular people and associated them with distressing meetings. Bronson reserves the term "fearful" for these cases and suggests that there may be three sorts of negative reaction to strangers. The youngest babies may be *distressed* by sudden physical approach or banging noise, while at five to six months a baby may feel *wariness* based on the unfamiliarity of a stranger as compared with an increasingly strongly held inner picture of his mother. Later in the first year, when the baby has a wider range of experiences and the intellectual capacity to remember them and to develop expectations for people's behavior, sheer unfamiliarity probably becomes less important, and *some* babies will develop particular fears grounded on particular associations.

Bronson believes that a further finding from his study supports the claim that what can cause fear changes sharply in the second half of the first year. It was not possible to predict, from the reaction of an individual baby at six and a half months to the approach of a stranger, the way in which he would react to the same situation at nine months. At the later age a few babies cried immediately because, Bronson thinks, the particular stranger in the study brought to mind earlier frightening associations. Physiological measures confirm the general picture of a qualitative change between five and nine months in the way babies react to strange situations. In a study by John Campos and others, nine-month-olds showed increased heartrates when a stranger approached in their mother's absence; but five-month-olds showed a decrease in heartrate. Recall that Sroufe's study found marked changes between six months and ten months, both in babies' behavior and in changes in heartrate in reaction to new situations.

There is, then, a profound shift that occurs when the child begins to recognize his mother's absence and to miss her presence in a new way. This indeed qualifies as a developmental milestone. But whether we should talk of "fear of strangers" as a milestone seems much more dubious. For a start, many babies in real life outside the laboratory never react to strangers in a way that could be called fearful. They show wariness, and a new caution, but no negative reaction. And this point is now at last being noticed by psychologists in laboratories. Many recent studies (for example, by Harriet Rheingold and Carol Eckerman[5]) comment on the infrequency of fearful responses to strange people and the inconsistency in the age when they appear, if they do. In Sroufe's study of the reaction of ten-month-olds, it was much more common for the babies to smile at the stranger and offer him a toy than it was to cry. It is clear that new situations and strange people interest and arouse babies, and careful observation suggests they activate both fearful and pleasurable feelings. This careful attention to the different signs of coyness, ambivalence, and so forth, that babies show in different situations is an essential step to take before we can solve the problems of understanding changes in children's reactions to strange situations. Which emotional state develops depends, among other things, on the setting, its familiarity, the presence of friendly family, and of course on how the strange people behave toward the baby and his parent. The complexity of the baby's response leads us to a third issue.

One system or several? We cannot treat the way a child reacts to a new situation, or indeed to any situation, as the reflection of just one set of feelings, such as fear. We know that as
adults we react in more complicated ways, and there is plenty of
evidence to support the idea that babies do so too. In one study
by Inge Bretherton and Mary Salter Ainsworth, 85 percent of the
babies showed friendly, "affiliative" behavior as well as fearful
behavior.[6] In a way, the concentration of research on the "fear
of strangers" phenomenon, and the mental processes underpin-
ning it, has blinded us to the richness and complexity of a child's
reaction to the unfamiliar. What is needed is much more precise
observation of children's behavior in different situations, before
we can decide whether it is reasonable to talk of two "systems"
of emotions in operation—the fear system and the affiliative—or
even of four, as Bretherton and Ainsworth suggest (exploration,
fear-wariness, attachment, and affiliation).

Survival values. A fourth issue arises from considering
whether it makes sense to think of the child's fear as part of a single behavioral system; it concerns the way in which we interpret
the adaptive value (that is, the importance for a baby's survival)
of different distress and fear reactions. People have tended to
describe fear as if it were part of a single system because of their
interest in the evolutionary value of behavior. It makes good
simple sense to interpret much of the behavior described here as
behavior adapted to the avoidance of danger—crying, with its
powerful effect on the parent, is an obvious example. The fact
that new situations produce both positive and negative feelings
is also easy to interpret as adaptive, since it is so important for a
creature both to find out about the world and to avoid its dan-
gers. We could also think about the adaptive value of children's
behavior when distressed as part of a "comforting system"—a
group of ways with which a child copes with upsetting or stressful events—turning away, crying, clinging, and, especially in the
second half of the first year, using a comfort object.

Paralleling the profound change in the quality of the baby's
attachment to his mother during the second half of the first year,
we find a new sort of attachment to the objects the baby asso-
ciates with comfort and security. It may be the bottle he takes to

bed, a fluffy blanket, a pacifier, or his own thumb—the source of comfort varies, but what seems common to all children is the intensity and persistence of their attachments, often for two or three years. The comfort such objects provide is very direct; they are in fact usually objects that are suckable or strokable, and when the children use them in moments of anxiety or tiredness the effects of sucking or stroking seem to parallel the effects of the continuous stimulation we see in very young babies. The rhythmic stimulation has a physically calming and sometimes soporific effect. In some cases children even use this effect to withdraw from painful or upsetting situations. But it is also important to notice how much the comforting effect of these objects depends on the significance the child attributes to them. The mere presence of the tattered blanket can transform the child's behavior. It enables him to tolerate and cope with situations that may otherwise fill him with anxiety. By no means do all children become attached to objects in this way, but if some particular object does become associated with security and comfort in the second half of the first year, this object takes on great importance for a long time and continues to be a source of comfort when the child has become a far more sophisticated creature. A nice illustration of this was reported by a mother of a twenty-month-old: the little boy, who was extremely lively and all over the place, had one day reduced his mother to tears of exhaustion and despair. As she sat crying on the bed, he ran to fetch his security blanket, which he habitually sucked in moments of tiredness or upset, and gave it to her, trying to push it into her mouth. He was grown up enough to recognize and sympathize with her distress, and yet the incident showed that his blanket was still a powerful source of comfort for him.

DO INDIVIDUAL DIFFERENCES PERSIST?

Does the baby who is very fretful in the early days go on being particularly miserable? To what extent do the differences between babies in the relative degree of their distress, wariness, or fearfulness remain consistent over time? There is one big problem in looking for continuities in personality differences. Take the baby who cries a great deal at four or five months: what should we look for when he is three years old, as a continuation of this four-month-old behavior? We know that crying means different things at different ages, and we would not necessarily expect the baby who cries a lot at five months to be the three-year-old who is always in tears. In fact, one study by Michael Lewis found that the babies who cried a great deal at six months were not the ones who cried at five years old.[7] They were, however, very aggressive in frustrating situations. Thus the problem is that, when we find differences between babies in irritability or wariness or other sorts of behavior, it is not at all clear what we should look for at a later age.

We have seen that where we find discontinuities in individual differences in behavior, as children grow up, these may help us to understand how and why the behavior has changed. Bronson's finding that there was little connection between individual patterns of wariness to strangers at six months and fear of a particular stranger at nine months fitted well with the idea that by nine months the child's emotional reaction had changed in character.

Earlier we saw that there is good evidence that babies differ markedly in irritability in the earliest days. How persistent are these differences over the first few months? Bronson made an attempt to relate each mother's descriptions of her child's reactions at one month to observations of the child's reaction to a stranger at four, six, and nine months. He asked the mothers whether their one-month-old babies cried a lot and how they had reacted to being bathed. In addition, he observed the degree of startle the babies showed to the sudden movement of an opening parasol. The results showed that babies who at one month cried more, and cried when being bathed, were frightened of the parasol and were more likely to be wary of a stranger at four months. Beyond this point, though, the connection did not seem to hold.

Some interesting connections were found by Kagan between the responses of four-month-olds to masks they had never seen before and the reactions of the same babies to being separated from their mothers in the laboratory at eight months and thirteen months. The four-month-olds who became restless and irritable when shown the masks were more likely to be fretful at eight and thirteen months, and were more likely to cry when separated from their mothers.

In this study Kagan was interested in trying to relate these differences in restlessness, and in response to the masks, to the intellectual development of the children. We know that the babies who show wariness to a strange situation have developed the ability to distinguish the familiar from the unfamiliar. Does this mean that individual differences in the age at which wariness develops, or in the intensity of the baby's fear response, are related to differences in other aspects of intellectual development in the first year? There is no clear answer to this question. Most studies suggest that there is no relation between the age at which children first show wariness and measures of their intellectual development. This could mean that the level of understanding demanded is so low that all the babies studied have it. Or it could reflect the fact that the fear response used in most studies is too unreliable and inconsistent. But there was one especially interesting finding in Kagan's study. Among the four-month-olds, twenty-one were extremely fretful when they were repeatedly shown the masks. These twenty-one were matched with children of the same sex and social class who never fretted when faced with the masks, and the pairs were compared at eight, thirteen, and twenty-seven months. No differences were found at eight months, but at thirteen and twenty-seven months, the girls who had been very irritable at four months showed signs of being intellectually precocious. They looked longer at discrepant events, played in a less stereotyped way at thirteen months, and were more talkative at twenty-seven months. We cannot of course say whether it is the child's particular temperament or intellectual ability that underlies this sort of continuity or whether it is just that her environment had not changed. It could be, for instance, that the four-month-old restlessness was the result of a very responsive, interested, and intrusive parenting style, and that this same style tended to produce children who were talkative and sophisticated as two year olds. This is an issue we will return to later, when we discuss how different patterns of parenting relate to fretfulness and separation anxiety.

CRYING INTENTIONALLY

One of the greatest changes in the child's signaling of distress during the first year comes with the development of deliberate crying. We have noted that when the newborn cries he has a disturbing effect on the adults around him, without being aware of the effect or being able to use it intentionally. During the early months, crying comes to be used as a controllable device for getting attention and help; it is quite clear with a one-year-old that crying is just one of many signals for directing adult attention to his needs and requests. Tracing the development of this intentional control presents many problems. The major difficulty is that, if we are to decide when the means to an end are being used intentionally, we have to be able to distinguish the means from the end. It is clear enough that a baby wants a particular toy when we watch him try a number of different ways to get it. But it is not so easy to tell from observation that a baby has begun to use crying deliberately to get adult attention and contact. Therefore most of the observations that help us to understand the beginnings of intentional behavior have been made in the context of the baby's play with objects.

Piaget noted that when his own child, Laurent, was around three months old he began to make a conscious connection between his own actions and particular events that followed.[8] He discovered that pulling on his father's watch chain, to which toys were attached, resulted in the toys' movement. After careful observation and experiment, Piaget became sure that around this age his children were able to distinguish the means from the end or goal they achieved. In these sequences the child was deliberately repeating an action that had had a particular effect. Although Piaget was sure that the child had distinguished the means by which he had achieved a particular end—such as making the toys swing—he only repeated the sequence of actions in this particular situation. It is not until the second half of the first year that we see the child definitely dissociating means from ends, when we find him applying means he has used in one situation to try to achieve the same end in quite a different one. In fact, bare descriptions of three- and four-month-old babies repeating sequences of actions could well be interpreted as evidence of conditioned responses; there would be nothing special in showing that the baby was repeating an action that led to a desired result, since we know that babies learn to do this at a much younger age. Whether we agree to call Laurent's action in shaking his father's watch chain "intentional" depends on how much we would agree that Laurent was making a conscious connection between shaking the chain and getting the result. Piaget stressed that, when a child pulls a chain in order to move the toys, he is carrying out a much more sophisticated behavioral pattern than when he simply grasps an object that he sees. He called it "a rudiment of intention." He also drew attention to the way Laurent varied the way he pulled the chain, watching the different effects he produced: "On seeing the child's expression it is impossible not to deem this gradation intentional."

Beyond these examples, where the child repeats actions over and over again to achieve the same effect, there are more complicated situations, where we can see what the child is trying to achieve and can observe his efforts to find some new way of reaching the goal. Piaget observed here his child's attempts to reach his watch when he put his own hand in the way, and noted the point at which the child first pushed away the hand deliberately in order to reach the watch; this happened at around the eighth month.

The child's growing sense of the effects of his signals on adults develops a further sophistication toward the end of the first year. This is the stage at which the baby begins to realize that adults can be used to provide help in the play with objects, and that objects can be used to gain adult attention. Look at the distinction made in Elisabeth Bates's study between the way a little girl, Carlotta, behaved with objects at eight to nine months and the way she behaved at eleven months.[9]

Observation 1 (before 10 months)
   In an effort to obtain a box that mother is holding in her arms, Carlotta pulls at the arms, pushes her whole body against the floor, and approaches the box from several angles. Yet during the entire sequence she never looks at her mother's face.

Observation 2 (at 11 months 22 days)
   Carlotta, unable to pull a toy cat out of the adult's hand, sits back up straight, looks the adult intently in the face, and then tries once again to pull the cat. The pattern is repeated three times . . . The interruption of an object play sequence to look towards the adult permits us to infer that the child now understands the potential role of the adult.

By observing the behavior of children with objects in this way we can map out the increasing power and elaboration of the baby's intentional behavior. However, the emphasis on the development of this kind of behavior with objects may be a little misleading for our understanding of the beginnings of intentional behavior in general. We cannot conclude that, because the nine-month-old is unaware of the potential role of adults in helping with the world of objects, he is unaware of how his own signals can influence adults. It seems in fact very likely that a nine-month-old baby has been aware for many weeks that his signals of distress are often followed by adult attention and he has been putting his awareness into practice. For the child to make this conscious connection between his own crying and adult reaction may well parallel the sort of understanding described of Piaget's son, at three or four months. There are good *a priori* reasons, about which both those in the psychoanalytic and behavioral traditions would agree, to expect that the capacity to act intentionally is developed in the most distressful and significant interactions, especially those with parents. We will see in a later chapter that in one area of intellectual development that has been studied carefully—the understanding that things and people continue to exist even when the baby cannot see them—most babies begin to understand about the permanence of their mother well before they understand object permanence. This means that it is important to study the development of intentional actions as they occur in the child's interactions with his family and not solely with objects—an exceptionally difficult area of study.

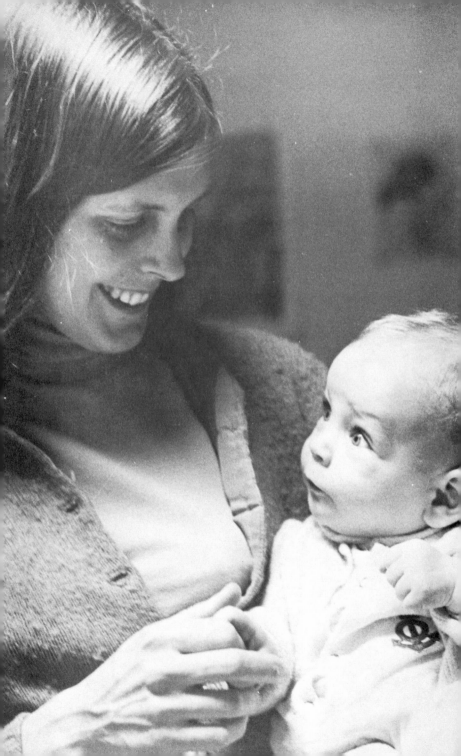

5 / Child and Parent in the Early Months

People studying the growth of a child's personality and the development of his social relationships have taken rather different attitudes to the part played by distress and comfort. Although most psychologists see the early exchange between mother and baby as very important for the way the relationship between the two develops, their views on why and how this is important vary widely, and lead to rather different recommendations concerning care for babies. How well do these ideas fit with what we know about the effects of different patterns of care for babies? In this chapter we will look briefly at some of the questions and at some recent research on different patterns of care.

THE PSYCHOANALYTIC APPROACH

Most theories of social development in children have grown out of the psychoanalytic concern with the importance of the mother-child relationship as the prototype of all later relationships. The psychoanalytic tradition, which goes back to the work of Freud, focuses mainly on emotional disorientation in adult life and on its causes. The theories, assumptions, and conclusions of psychoanalysts vary greatly. For our purposes we do not need any detailed account of the variations, but it is a matter of considerable importance that much of the most sensitive scientific work on distress and comfort in infancy has been either initiated by psychoanalysts or strongly influenced by their thinking. The central focus of psychoanalysis is upon the emotional condition of children and adults, and it has provided a whole dimension of thinking about issues on which the other traditions in psychology have few resources to contribute. The various psychoanalytical schools of thought take rather different views of the earliest stages of this first "love" relationship, but all of them agree that the course of the relationship with the mother and father has a great influence on the way in which the child's personality develops, on his feelings about himself, on his later personal relationships, and his ability to cope with everyday problems. How do psychoanalytic theorists view the role played by the early experience of distress, and the comfort provided by the parent, in this development?

Many follow Freud's suggestion that the origin of the child's relationship with his mother lies in the sensations with which she provides him in the feeding situation. According to Anna Freud, what becomes associated with the mother is the "blissful experience of satisfaction and relief" produced by the reduction of tension when the child feeds. The relationship with the mother develops as a secondary consequence of the way she provides relief from hunger and thirst. The baby's emotional dependence on his mother grows out of his physical need to reduce the discomfort of hunger. There are many difficulties faced by theories of this kind, which try to explain the growth of social relationships as secondary to the gratification of such drives as hunger and thirst. But I will mention here only some of the ways in which the parental role of comforting has been viewed.

The psychoanalytic focus is on what the infant is experiencing or feeling at the early stages. This is imagined and described in varied ways in the different psychoanalytic theories, and these differences in the imagined experience are then seen to have special implications for the child's development. The descriptions are inevitably speculative, and since there can be no way of testing them, it would not be useful to enlarge on the differences here. We can note, however, that they all focus on an issue of great importance in development—the way in which the child begins to distinguish between himself and others. All the theorists agree that the experiences of pleasure and pain play a central part in this differentiation—but they focus in different ways on the stage at which the child shifts from narcissism to distinguishing himself from other people and to developing social relationships. One particular idea that will recur in our discussion of comfort and distress is the notion of the child's developing confidence and trust. Anna Freud and Therese Benedek see the development of the child's ability to wait for food instead of crying impatiently as indicating a major stride in development. When a child can manage this, he has gained a sense of confidence that his needs will be met. Therese Benedek sees this confidence providing an "emotional shelter" that enables the child to turn his attention away from his own needs and toward the environment. To Erik Erikson this basic trust means both that the child has learned to rely on the continuity of the providers in his world and that he now has some sense of mastery.[1]

All analysts see maternal love and comfort as vital to human development. However, they link very different elements in the care a baby receives to the differences in individual personalities later. If we look at case histories, it is clear that for many analysts the way an infant has progressed through the early months is seen as central in determining his character and personality as an adult. Differences in caregiving and early experiences can lead to the child's becoming fixated (stuck) at any point in what is postulated as a standard sequence of psychosexual development. This fixation is thought to influence not only the type of person with whom he, as an adult, will become emotionally involved but also the sort of behavior he will show toward his "attachment object" (how he will treat those with whom he becomes involved). For instance, deprivation at the earliest "oral" stage of infancy, when the baby's interests are centered on sucking and mouthing activities, is often seen as linked to later feelings of pessimism, depressive tendencies, and demanding, sadistic, or aggressive qualities.

Writers such as Sibylle Escalona and René Spitz clearly feel that the mother can help or hinder the child's progress through these stages. But many psychoanalytic writers are not concerned with the details of parental response to the child in the earliest months. They write generally about the emotions within the family rather than specifically about patterns of care and parental response. Among those who do discuss the way parents can affect the child's development, the views range from Freud's hard line on gratification and comfort to the very different attitude of John Bowlby, which we will look at subsequently. Freud himself felt that a child could be spoiled by too much gratification and would, as a result, both demand and miss gratification more: "The undesirable result of 'spoiling' a small child is to magnify the danger of losing . . . [his] protection against . . . helplessness . . . It therefore encourages the individual to remain in the state of childhood."[2] He also put considerable emphasis on the importance of frustration and "unpleasure" in forming personality. Spitz, too, stressed the importance of frustration and specified the infant "diseases" that arise from particular maternal attitudes: three-month colic, for example, he linked to maternal overpermissiveness. As we will see, there is great contrast between this view and that of other writers within the psychoanalytic tradition.

THE SOCIAL-LEARNING APPROACH

To the social-learning theorists, whose ideas are derived from the basic psychoanalytic concern with the importance of the child's relationship with the mother, the individual ways that caregivers respond to a child's actions, signals, and requests are of central importance. One group believes that the development of a child's social behavior can be understood by considering the rewards and punishments (the reinforcers) for various kinds of behavior that he has experienced throughout infancy. This suggests that what a child enjoys and hence seeks in social relationships will vary from family to family. The child who is cuddled and rocked will develop a definite wish for physical contact and closeness. The mother of another child may consistently respond to him with more distant exchanges—such as looks, talking, or smiles—and he in turn will develop a more distant style of interaction. Depending on how their own behavior is responded to, children will develop different patterns of behavior with others. Some will become clinging, expecting a great deal of attention, approval, comment, and so on.

There are three points of interest to note here. First, those items of the child's behavior that are most likely to be responded to and reinforced by the mother's attention are indeed expressions of distress and requests for attention. So the way in which she responds to his distress is particularly important. Social-learning theorists have emphasized that the mother's immediate response on hearing the child cry gives the child a sense of effective power; it is thus important in developing a sense of mastery.

A second interesting feature is that the pattern of parental response to the child's distress influences how firmly established his behavior becomes. It has been shown in learning experiments that the responses that are most firmly established, and the most resistant to being altered, are not those which are responded to 100 percent of the time, but those which are responded to irregularly. Real-life schedules of response to a crying child will of course certainly be intermittent, and it is plainly of great practical importance that this actual pattern of response to crying is just what will make the child more likely to cry. Many writers do not appear to consider any particular response from the mother as necessarily more important or effective than any other; physical contact, for example, is by no means always emphasized as important. What matters is that the mother's response follows quickly on the baby's action, so that over a period he links the two in his mind. Contact with the mother means not simply physical contact; Walters and Parke in particular stress the importance of the baby's watching and attending to others as a way of maintaining contact with them.[3]

A third particularly useful feature of the social-learning approach is that it also emphasizes the baby's behavior in its important reinforcing effects on the mother. Each mother-baby pair develops a particular way of interacting together, a particular pattern of attachment. This is an idea that has been well understood, and carefully studied for many years, by ethologists looking at animals and birds. It is a little surprising that it has only recently been greeted with interest as a new approach to development by those studying children.

HOW DIFFERENCES BETWEEN MOTHERS AFFECT BABIES

How well do these ideas fit with the results of the recent studies of babies with their parents and caregivers?

Louis Sander's fine study shows very clearly the way in which a baby's crying behavior is influenced from the earliest days by whoever looks after him.[4] He studied the patterns of crying and sleeping in babies brought up by two nurses who acted as foster mothers. After ten days in a nursery, each baby was transferred to a room where he was looked after individually, twenty-four hours a day, by one of the two nurses, Nurse A or Nurse B. The babies transferred to the care of Nurse B showed an abrupt decrease in crying from the high levels they had shown in the nursery, while those who were transferred to the care of Nurse A showed a much less definite change (see Figure 3).

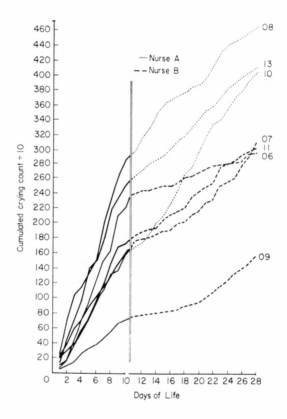

3. *Cumulative crying counts in seven babies reared in the nursury during the first 10 days of life and then cared for either by Nurse A or Nurse B on days 11 to 28.*

Now there are two different points to think about in these results. First, according to the social-learning theory, the more a baby is responded to the more he will cry. In fact Nurse A did respond more quickly and more frequently than Nurse B, and the babies in her care cried most—just what the theorists would have predicted. However, the greatest amount of crying went on in the nursery where the babies spent their first ten days, and it is likely that here the attention they received when they cried was both slower and less frequent. Over the first few days it seems that a slow response to crying may well lead to more rather than less crying. In the nursery the babies were looked after by many different nurses, and the care must have been ill adjusted to the needs of the individual baby. This individual attention is thought to be very important by Sander: he stressed that Nurse B was particularly effective at soothing and calming her babies because in some way her care was more sensitive—she took more account of the individual differences between babies than Nurse A did. This notion of sensitivity toward the baby brings us to Bowlby's ideas on the attachment between mother and baby, and the part played by early comfort and distress in this relationship.[5]

ATTACHMENT THEORY

John Bowlby, in his theory of attachment, stresses the fact that the baby's signals of distress and the mother's comforting response to them have a biological function. Crying and the mother's response are seen as one part of a system of behavior bonding mother and child closely together—a system that has the biological function of protecting the young from predators. Bowlby emphasizes the way in which the behavior that attaches mother and child resembles that of the higher apes, pointing out the survival value of systems that ensure close proximity and contact between infant and mother during the long period of immaturity of all the higher apes. Among the apes and monkeys, the newborn is always in close contact with the mother's body; he may maintain this contact by clinging and sucking the nipple, or he may be supported by the mother's hold. As the young ape or monkey grows up, he begins to spend time away from his mother. The changes in the relative time spent close to the mother, and the member of the pair who is responsible for maintaining proximity, has been the subject of detailed research by Robert Hinde. At any sign of danger or upset, the young will move immediately to the mother, and the mother to the young. Bowlby and Mary Ainsworth and Sylvia Bell use this "spatial" link as a hall mark of attachment, a "set-goal" of being close to the mother that will vary in different circumstances and with the age of the infant:

> The behavioural hallmark of attachment is seeking to gain and to maintain a certain degree of proximity to the object of attachment, which ranges from close physical contact under some circumstances to interaction or communication across some distance under other circumstances. Attachment behaviours are behaviours which promote proximity or contact. In the human infant these include active proximity- and contact-seeking behaviours such as approaching, following, and clinging, and signalling behaviours such as smiling, crying, and calling.[6]

When the attachment system is intensely activated, by fear or danger, physical contact between infant and mother will be necessary to bring attachment seeking to an end. At lower levels of activation, contact over distance may be enough—a look and smile may reassure.

Bowlby sees the young baby's crying as one of five built-in signals; these form part of the system by which, with the appropriate response of the mother, physical closeness is ensured. Not only is the baby's behavior built in, but the mother is seen as genetically programmed to respond to this behavior—though an overlay of learned responses may interfere with her "natural' response (just as they have with her "natural" habitat). In emphasizing protection rather than feeding as the essential biological function of mothering, Bowlby uses Harry Harlow's experiments with rhesus monkeys as supporting evidence. Harlow reared infant monkeys with inanimate surrogate mothers made either from wire mesh or covered with toweling. He showed that the infant rhesus sought proximity and contact more often from the towel "mother," who provided contact and comfort, than from the wire "mother," who provided food. The baby monkeys in fact became intensely attached to the towel mother. As Harlow pointed out, this was a finding that directly contradicted the idea that the baby became attached to the mother because he associated her with reduction in hunger or thirst.

Harlow's rhesus experiments provide a compelling parallel to the observations on the important effect of the mother's presence or absence on the way the human child explores or responds to the presence of a stranger. He showed that, once an attachment had been made to a surrogate mother, the baby monkey was able to use the mother as a source of comfort when alarmed by a fearful stimulus and as a base from which he could explore. As we will see, young children behave in a strikingly similar way. More powerful evidence that the attachment between a human mother and her baby has much in common with that in nonhuman primates has come from the studies of the dramatic effects on young primates who are separated from their mothers. The young monkeys showed reactions of great distress and then depression, and these reactions bear very strong resemblances to the reactions of children separated from their parents.

Charles Kaufman comments on the appearance of the pigtail macaque monkey infant after a day of separation from its mother, when it begins to show a severe depression (Figure 4). "When the face could be seen it had the appearance of dejection and sadness Darwin described and believed 'to be universally and instantly recognized as that of grief.' "[7]

Although the object of the various kinds of attachment behavior is closeness between the mother and infant (in the sense that this is what brings them to an end), the particular actions involved may be quite different with infants of different ages within one species, and may be quite different in different species. Thus a human child shows attachment behavior in the first weeks of life by crying and, at the end of the first year, by following, stretching out his arms, and clinging; among the nonhuman primates, the differing ways of life and habitat of the various species mean that they may show different behavior. The rhesus monkey clings from the first day, the baby chimpanzee is carried. Once a baby (of whatever species) is in contact with the mother, many different experiences will reinforce his desire to be close to her.

In Bowlby's view, then, crying and the mothers' prompt response to it play an important part in the growth of attachment. He argues that within the nuclear family every child will become

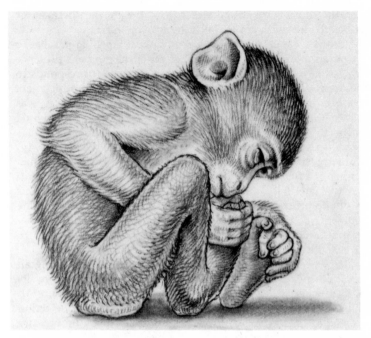

4. *Depressed pigtail infant.*

attached, but that the *quality* of the attachment will depend on the sensitivity of the mother. The mother's prompt and appropriate response to the child's distress—the response to which she is seen as "biologically attuned" as a member of her species—is taken as one feature of the sensitivity that is critical for the development of a stable and happy relationship.

But is it easy to pick out sensitive mothers? In Sander's study of the two foster-mother nurses, Nurse B was seen as sensitive because she was more effective at soothing and calming her babies. However, if we are going to use the notion of sensitivity in response to crying, we must remember that even in the newborn period there may well be great differences not only between mothers but also between babies—in what makes them cry and what stops them. We have not yet much idea of what the range of these differences might be, but we will have to find some way of assessing how consolable babies are before we can compare mothers in their skill at soothing.

Bowlby's idea of sensitive mothering does assume a neat fit between the needs of the baby and the performance of the mother. But it is always so simple to decide what an appropriate response is? Appropriate for what? Nurse A in Sander's study was much less effective at soothing her crying babies. But the babies in her care did in fact sleep longer. How are we to judge what is better for the baby—a quick response and a great deal of sleep, or a more wakeful life with fewer distressful episodes? Sander himself warns against judging prematurely. And from the parents' point of view, there may well be occasions in the early weeks when it is not at all clear why the baby is crying, or what the most appropriate response would be.

DIFFERENCES BETWEEN BABIES

We have seen that how long babies cry, and how frequently, is very much influenced by how they are looked after, even in the first week. But what about the effects of babies on their parents? We know that newborns differ a great deal in their irritability and in their consolability. This great range of individual variation continues over the early months. Freda Rebelsky examined how much babies cried from two weeks to thirteen weeks by a system of automatic recording.[8] Ten babies wore small recording devices for one twenty-four-hour period every fortnight; the recorders started automatically whenever the babies cried. Over this period how much each baby cried in his two-weekly recording varied considerably; but the difference between babies was much greater than this variation within each baby's score. When the total amount of crying for all recordings was averaged, one baby's average was as much as sixty-four minutes in twenty-four hours, while another's was only seven minutes. Again, great individual variation was found in the periods within the day when crying occurred: one baby cried, on average, during five hours of the twenty-four, and another during twelve.

Of course this sort of information does not tell us how far continuing differences between the babies stem from continuing differences in their irritability, or how far they reflect consistent differences in the mothers rather than in the babies. What do we know about the links between crying and the way the baby has been cared for, after the newborn period? Is a mother who is very responsive in the early weeks still very responsive by the end of the first year? And does a mother who responds very quickly encourage crying, or does she reassure the baby so that he cries less in the future? The two theoretical approaches that I have mentioned, the social-learning theory and the attachment theory, would give rather different answers here. According to attachment theory, we would probably expect that the most responsive mother, the one who provides her baby with the prompt appropriate response to his signal of distress, would develop a happy relationship with a baby who is contented and satisfied and who cries little. According to social-learning theory, the baby who receives prompt attention may well cry more frequently in the future, since he has been rewarded by attention on the earlier occasions of crying.

The most comprehensive study of these questions has been made in Baltimore by Mary Ainsworth and Sylvia Bell.[9] They found that babies whose crying was ignored early on tended to cry more frequently and more persistently later in the first year and that, after the first six months, this persistent crying discouraged the mothers from responding. The researchers suggested too that the mothers who had responded quickly to their babies had children who were more likely to be advanced in "communication skills," as measured by comparing the range of facial expression in each baby. Further studies on individual differences in the security of the relationship between child and mother (studies we will be looking at in the next chapter) completed a picture in which the sensitive and prompt response of the mother was found to promote a harmonious relationship with a child who was content, obedient, secure, and competent. These results fit very well with attachment theory, and with the idea of the mother biologically programmed to respond immediately to her baby. Indeed, these psychologists see insensitive mothers who do not respond promptly as "going against nature," and they attribute the difficulties the mothers have with their demanding ambivalent children largely to the erosion of a natural relationship, erosion produced by anxiety about spoiling.

But results from other studies do not match this neat picture. Some suggest that the more prompt the mother's response, the more frequently the baby cries in later weeks. In our Cambridge study we also found that a mother's response to her baby's crying depended very much on how generally irritable he was at the time. If we had been looking for an index of sensitivity, this response to crying would have been misleading, since some mothers of fretful babies were not running quickly to attend to them when they cried, although they were loving and attentive in other ways.

Clearly there is a great deal of work to be done before we can make any simple rule of thumb about the consequences of a particular pattern of response to crying in the early weeks. What is extremely clear is the need for one thing: to take account of individual differences in baby irritability early on and, for another, to be careful not to treat measures of the mother's response as if they were unaffected by the particular characteristics of the baby she is looking after.

The difficulty in untangling the effects of mother on baby, and of baby on mother, are illustrated by the findings of a study of slightly older children by Alison Clarke-Stewart.[10] In this study thirty-six mother-child pairs were observed when the children were eleven, fourteen, and seventeen months old. The results from her sample suggested that mothers who respond promptly to distress tend to have children who are among the least fretful. However, when her results for boys and results for girls were examined separately, it was found that the most *and* the least fretful girls tended to have mothers who were very responsive to their signals of distress. Support is here, then, for the predictions of both social-learning theorists and attachment theorists.

Nor was there clear evidence in this study that the mother's responsiveness influenced the baby's irritability at a later date or that the child's level of irritability affected the mother's response to the baby's distress at a later date. But Clarke-Stewart did find another relationship: The mothers whose children had looked and "talked" to them a great deal at eleven months had become less rejecting and more responsive to the children's distress and demands by seventeen months. Psychologists have at last managed to show in objective terms something that parents and those who care for children have felt for a long time—children can have a very positive "turning-on" effect on those who look after them.

NEW DIRECTIONS

In talking about these studies I have contrasted the views of social-learning theorists and attachment theorists in a way that presents a somewhat overdramatic picture of the differences in the way psychologists study interaction. The framework within which most recent research has been carried out retains features of both approaches. For instance, in the study of the earliest social interactions we have recently learned a great deal about the capacity of babies from birth to *learn* about features of their environment and to adapt their behavior accordingly. But we have also discovered that babies are predisposed to learn particular features of their environment. Babies are especially sensitive, for instance, to sounds that fall within the frequency range of the human female voice, and they are particularly interested in looking at objects that have features in common with the human face. These findings plainly emphasize the great importance of the explicitly biological style of understanding which attachment theory has alerted people to. Both approaches are important in understanding the baby's powers of learning, though, and the constraints on what he is likely to learn.

Take the following observation: a six-week-old baby is crying in his crib. His mother comes to pick him up and holds him close, gently patting him. The baby stops crying, calms down. She holds him a little away now, face to face, and talks to him smiling. He gazes back intently and begins to coo. The features of this sequence that particularly excite researchers now unite both the learning aspects stressed by the social-learning theorists and the "meshing" of mother and baby behavior emphasized by the attachment approach—the close fit between expression of need and provision of comfort.

We are beginning to realize that this early exchange between mother and child has a place of great importance in the development of the child's understanding and powers of communication, in the slowly developing awareness of the other person. Close analysis of such interactions can tell us much about the baby's built-in capabilities for social behavior and his intense interest in people, can show the delicate turn-taking and timing already evident in the interlocking of looks and cooing, and how these in turn lead on to reciprocal interaction at a more complex level. The way in which mother and child learn to read each other's intentions is a focus of great interest to psychologists studying the beginnings of language. And they have stressed the importance of the occasions when mother and baby both pay attention to the same thing and when the baby comes to recognize that this is happening. This obviously takes many months to develop, and most research has fastened on the play and games between mother and child as the central ground on which the growth of this mutual focus and awareness can take place. It certainly seems possible that a mother's search to find out what her baby wants when he is distressed—her attempts to discover what is bothering him—and their mutual relief when she manages to find it can play an important part in this process. Whether it is a search for a particular cause of distress, or a search for a distraction that both mother and child can attend to together, this joint attention appears when the baby most needs and wants adult presence and response—when his awareness of the adult reaction to his signals will be at its most intense and perhaps at its most sensitive. It should not surprise us that some psychoanalytic writers should have stressed the close relationship of intellectual growth with emotional development.

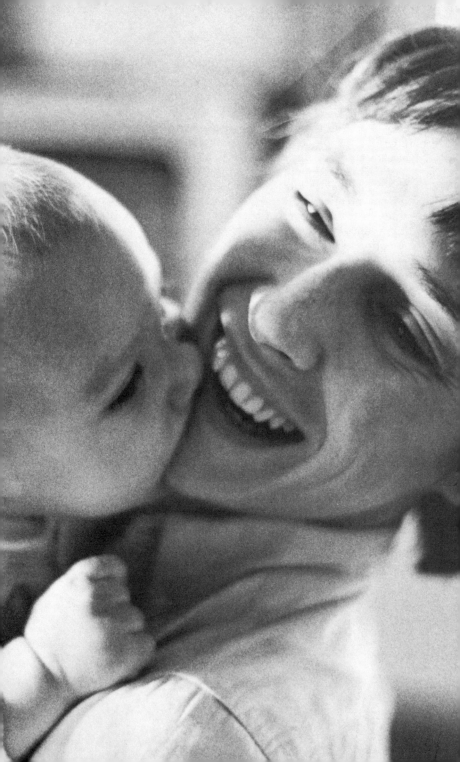

6 / Crying, Comfort, and Attachments

How do children's experiences of distress and comfort affect their relationship with their parents? When we looked at the Baltimore study of crying and maternal responsiveness, we saw that the way the mother responded to the baby's crying seemed important not just in influencing how much he cried, but also in they way the attachment relationship developed between them. Looking at the question makes us think about how relationships do in fact differ and about what the origins of these differences might be. These are central problems to psychologists today, and the work on distress highlights some of the most interesting advances, and some of the most intractable theoretical difficulties, in our understanding of early relationships.

Researchers looking in detail at the first relationships that babies form have reported differences in the age at which they first become attached to people, differences in the numbers of people to whom they become attached, differences in the intensity or quality of the relationships. What do we know about the factors underlying these differences? In what way is the experience of comfort important?

DIFFERENCES IN ATTACHMENT

In one of the first studies of attachment, by Rudolph Schaffer and Peggy Emerson, the baby's protesting response to everyday separations, such as being left outside a shop, or alone in a room at home, or to being put down after being held, was used as an index of attachment.[1] In this study, the time at which attachments to specific people were first noticed ranged from twenty-two weeks of age to fifteen months. But others have set the mile-stone earlier. Ainsworth and Bell found that babies would cry when their mothers left the room as early as fifteen weeks and would certainly cry by thirty weeks. The age at which the babies first became attached to specific people apparently had nothing to do normally with the way their mothers had behaved toward them (though Schaffer has shown that children who have been temporarily in an institution may begin to show attachments at a slightly later age on their return home). Within the families so far studied, then, the way in which crying is treated in the first year does not seem to affect the age at which children show def-inite signs of being attached.

According to the idea that dependence grows out of the satis-faction of primary needs like hunger, it is clear that a child should show his first and most important attachment to the per-son responsible for feeding him when he is hungry, warming him when he is cold, giving him drink when he is thirsty. The results of a number of studies have shown that this is *not* what happens. One fifth of the people to whom the babies in Schaffer's and Emerson's study became attached took no part at all in their physical care. Rather, the babies formed relationships with those people who were particularly responsive to their signals for at-tention and who initiated exchanges with them. This was by no means always the most available person: in fact, the amount of time the adult spent with the babies seemed unimportant. By eighteen months, in as much as a third of the sample it was the father to whom the baby seemed most attached.

Findings from studies of kibbutzim and of children in group care confirm this general picture: the child's early relationships are formed not necessarily with the person who relieves his pri-mary needs and discomforts, but with those who get involved with him in exciting and affectionate ways. In the kibbutzim, for instance, the children did not form attachments to the *metapelet* (caretaker) who looked after their needs during the day. With their parents, however, whom they saw for about two hours each evening, two hours of intense and loving interaction, the children formed attachments just as intense as those formed by American children brought up in ordinary families.

How often is an attachment formed toward the person who usually provides comfort when the child is distressed? By no means always. Indeed, experiments with animals suggest that in some circumstances attachments may develop to people or objects that cause distress. Michael Rutter writes that clinical experience indicates that the same may be true for man. "It is parental apathy and lack of response which appear more important as inhibitors of the child's attachment."[2] Very often, of course, it is the mother who relieves distress and meets the child's needs and also is involved in intense and exciting interactions with him.

It is quite clear that there are great differences in the extent to which children are upset by their mother's departure or absence, in the intensity with which they demand her attention, and in the intensity with which they enjoy her presence. What lies beneath these differences?

FORMS OF ATTACHMENT

Children express their attachment to their mothers in different ways. Some want lots of cuddling and holding, others like to stay close to their mothers and need a lot of attention but don't want to be held, others are happy wandering away from their mothers but are delighted by looks and "conversation." How much a particular child needs and requests these different sorts of contact will vary with the situation and with how he is feeling. This variation does not mean that the underlying relationship is unstable. Mary Ainsworth has suggested that we need to distinguish between the *expression of attachment* and the underlying *attachment bond*. She underlines the point that showing attachment—wanting to be near the mother, and so on—may be only one of the things a child wants to do. He may also, for instance, want to explore. It is an important distinction. In some circumstances a baby will try more often and harder to be close to his mother—when he is tired or frightened or in a new situation. But it is a distinction that leaves us with a considerable problem: if the expression of attachment varies despite the stability of the attachment "bond" itself, how can we identify the precise character of this bond?

Exploration, comfort, and staying close. The second problem in comparing differences in children's attachment to their parents is that the developing child is also an exploring and adventurous child. We know that children spend less and less time being physically close to and touching their mothers between the ages of one and three. But it would be absurd to assume that this decline in wanting to be close necessarily indicates a change in the depth of the relationship. The balance between exploring the world and maintaining safe contact is obviously one of great importance to the child, and there is richness and subtlety in the variations of balance enjoyed by different mother-child pairs, a range of communication and understanding that varies greatly in intensity and expression. If we used only physical distance between mother and child to measure their relationship, we would be missing a great deal. We have to realize too that the physical closeness of a mother may mean very different things in different relationships. In a study of two mother-child pairs from birth to twelve months, Sibylle Escalona and Helen Corman showed that while the presence of the mother had a marked effect on how both children behaved, it affected them in opposite ways. One child became more active and responsive in all areas of behavior; the other became less alert, less responsive and animated.

With the distinction between attachment as a relationship or bond and attachment behavior, Mary Ainsworth prefers to talk about the *security* of attachment rather than the *strength* of the bond: the securely attached child she sees as one who explores confidently and who "uses the mother as a base from which to explore." Now we know that a vital feature of the attachment relationship is the security a child feels in the presence of the person he is attached to, and a number of experiments have demonstrated that the presence of this person enables him to explore a new or strange situation. Ainsworth and Barbara Wittig observed one-year-olds in a series of situations: in a laboratory playroom with the mother, with the mother and a stranger, alone with the stranger, or entirely on their own. When the mother was present, the children explored the strange room and toys, checking now and then on their mother's presence. When she left the room, most of the children immediately stopped their explorations, tried to follow, and became upset. The presence of a stranger did not upset the children's explorations provided the mother was there. When the mother reappeared after the separation episode, most of the children rushed to be held or picked up. The way the children investigated and played, then, depended on how confident they were about their mother's availability.

There are parallel experiments by Harlow with rhesus monkeys which illustrate both how fear increases attachment behavior such as clinging, and how an attachment figure provides comfort for a distressed infant and gives him the confidence to explore. When a young monkey, who had been brought up on a cloth surrogate mother, was placed in a strange place, or presented with a toy bear, he immediately rushed to the "mother" and clung to it. After a little while, he began to relax and started to look at the frightening new situation. Then slowly he started to leave the mother and began to explore. If the "mother" was not present, the young monkey would show signs of continuing distress and would not investigate.

In general terms, then, the security provided by the person to whom the child is attached is an enormously important aspect of their relationship, as every parent knows. And the notion that there are individual differences in the way children can use the mother as a base from which to explore does make very good intuitive sense. Still it is important that we think very carefully about the measures of behavior we use to show this security, lest we be left with the problem of being unable to distinguish the poorly attached child, content to be physically separated from his mother, from the securely attached child who is exploring. Ainsworth's measures of security of attachment focus on the child's responses to everyday brief separations.

Separation protest. Attempts to measure the "bond" between mother and child have centered on the child's distress at separation from the mother. But this again presents many problems. Is the child who waits confidently and shows no distress when his mother leaves less strongly involved with her than the child who cries a great deal? This is really the same problem as the one posed by the exploring child. It is already clear that the way children respond to being separated from their mothers during an experiment in a laboratory does not relate closely to the way they react to everyday separations at home. Most twelve-month-olds showed less "separation distress" at home than in a laboratory situation, though on the other hand some of those who protested frequently at home showed no protest in the laboratory. Again, not all children are distressed at brief separations from their mother at home, although their very happy greetings on reunion make it clear that they have a real attachment to her.

Although laboratory studies give the impression that distress at separation is a common response, at home only a minority of the episodes where the mother leaves the room lead to crying or fussing. It is now clear that the distress a young child shows varies according to the child's age, the way the mother actually leaves the room (for instance, whether she speaks to him), and the familiarity of the situation. It also depends on his previous experience of separation. When a two-year-old is tested for a second time in a laboratory situation, he is more upset and anxious than he was on the first occasion. In sum, distress at separation depends very much on the particular situation, and it would be very misleading to see it, on its own, as a revealing index of the quality of the relationship between child and mother.

The origins of differences in distress at separation. How distressed a child becomes when he is separated from his mother is, then, difficult to use as a sign of the "quality" of the relationship between them. Given that differences between children upset at separation are difficult to interpret, it is not surprising that we do not get a simple answer to the origins of these individual differences.

Two different studies have given us two different stories. In their study of children in Glasgow, Schaffer and Emerson asked mothers at monthly intervals about their children's usual response to everyday separation situations, such as being left alone in a room at home, being put down after a cuddle, being left outside a shop, and being put to bed at night. There was no correlation between the degree of upset the child showed in these separations and the sex of the child, his position in the family, the mother's social class, and so on. But links were found with the mother's response to her baby's demands, with how much interaction there was between mother and baby, and with the way the baby protested at separation. The more responsive mothers had babies who protested more at separation. Schaffer stresses that these results tell us nothing of the *direction* of the cause and effect: "Do infants develop intense attachments because they have mothers who enjoy and foster this type of behavior? Or do infants force the mother to respond in certain ways by the urgency of their demands?"

Individual differences between babies are, as we have seen, very important in influencing how parents behave. We also know that genetic differences play an important part in differences in social behavior. Identical twins, for instance, are significantly more alike in their behavior than fraternal twins, who don't share identical genetic make-up. We find this even when we look at twin babies as young as eight or nine months old.

A significantly different picture of the origins of individual differences in distress at separation came from the Baltimore study of Ainsworth. The children who cried most when their mothers left the room were least likely to greet them in a happy way when they returned; they were most likely to react with crying or ambivalence. These were also the children who cried most frequently and longest during the observation as a whole, and were most likely to fuss when they were put down after being held. These observations give us a convincing picture of a difficult relationship between mother and child. And the children who were the most extreme in their crying and ambivalence were those whose mothers were rated as least sensitive and least responsive to their babies crying. The researchers felt that a mother, by being unresponsive to her child, has more effect on the baby's crying than vice-versa, and so they set the responsibility for the origins of the difficult relationship firmly on the mother's doorstep.

It is not easy to reconcile the results of the two studies. The findings of both make good sense in terms of our own human experience. If a child has had a relationship with a warm and responsive mother, it seems natural that he should particularly mind her absence. On the other hand, if he is generally anxious and insecure about his relationships, we would expect him to be more upset than others by any extra stress. It may be that there are different sorts of distress shown by children briefly separated from their families and that these sorts of upset have different origins. If a child is very distressed when his mother leaves him, is he missing her because their relationship is so rich and enjoyable, or is he generally an anxious child? It certainly seems likely that a simple label of "separation protest" masks wide differences in children's behavior, just as did the label "fear of strangers." The Baltimore study gives us a vivid picture of children who are insecure when their mothers leave them and ambivalent toward them when they are present; when we are thinking about the development of this difficult relationship, we must remember that many of the mother's actions that contribute to her sensitivity, as rated here, are already strongly influenced by the individual characteristics of her baby. So when we describe her sensitivity in this way we are really describing how this mother gets on with this particular baby.

It is important to remember that, in this discussion of the relation between a baby's anxious attachment and his response to his mother's leaving him, we have been thinking about only the everyday separations occurring in the home. There is no evidence that the intensity of a child's distress when he is separated from his mother in a hospital situation, or suffers a major separation lasting for days, is related to a previously difficult relationship with his mother. We look next at children's responses to these longer separations.

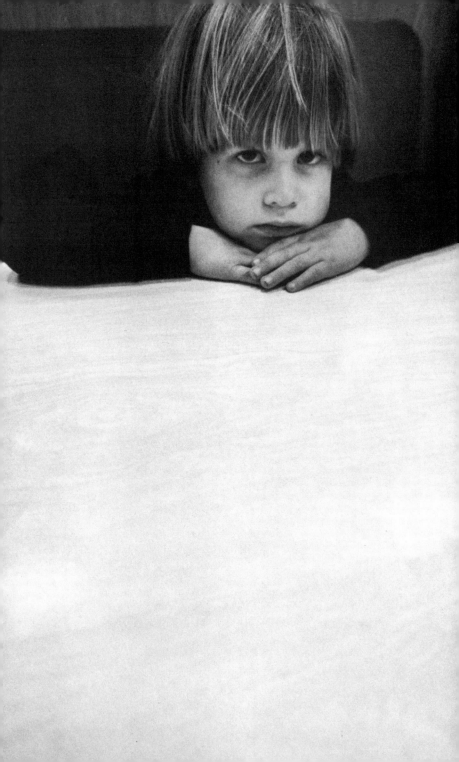

7 / The Response to Longer Separations

When young children have to spend time away from their families in residential care or in hospitals, nearly all of them show immediate distress. Very often this is followed by a period of apathetic misery, and for some children there is a later stage of apparent "detachment" from their parents. The intensity of the first distress stage has been vividly described in a study by Christoph Heinicke and Ilse Westheimer of ten children cared for in a residential nursery. The response of the children to the separation is summarized by John Bowlby:

> When the moment came for the parents to depart, crying or screaming was the rule. One child tried to follow her parents, demanding urgently where they were going, and finally had to be pushed back into the room by her mother. Another threw himself on the floor and refused to be comforted. Altogether eight of the children were crying loudly soon after their parents' departure. Bedtime was also an occasion for tears. The two who had not cried earlier screamed when put in a cot and could not be consoled. Some of the others whose initial crying had ceased broke into renewed sobs at bedtime. One little girl who arrived in the evening and was put straight to bed insisted on keeping her coat on, clung desperately to her doll, and cried "at a frightening pitch." Again and again having nodded off from sheer fatigue, she awoke screaming for Mummy.[1]

This picture of extreme distress has been confirmed by several studies, and it underlines how much the essence of the relationship between the parent and the young child is one of security. Children do, after all, very often enjoy new places if their parents are there. Looking at what will relieve the children's distress can be very revealing. First it can tell us about what is distressing the child—whether it is the separation, the strange environment, the disruption of the bond between the child and those he loves, or the lack of any friendly person he can attach himself to. But, second, it can tell us about the child's relationships with people other than his mother and the nature of those relationships. For instance, is the child's relationship with his mother special and different from his relationships with other members of his family?

We will look first very briefly at what can significantly modify the degree of distress a child suffers at being separated.

THE DEGREE OF DISTRESS

Temperament. There is a great variation in the way individual children respond to being separated and, although there have been few systematic studies of this, it does seem that there are some personality differences that have a clear effect on the child's response. Stacey and his colleagues found that children who were socially inhibited, or were aggressive and had difficulties making relationships with other adults or children, were most likely to be disturbed when admitted to hospital.[2]

Age and sex. We have seen the importance of the changes that take place over the first year in the baby's powers of understanding. This means that, before six or seven months of age, there is usually no sign of distress when babies are exposed to extended separation. Children admitted to hospital from the age of six months up to four or five years, however, usually show acute distress. It is possible, though far from certain, that boys are more disturbed by separation experiences than girls.

Previous experience of separation. If young children (or animals) have already had unhappy separation experiences, they seem more likely to be particularly upset by another separation. Recent experiments with rhesus monkeys show that long-term effects are greater when the baby monkeys have experienced two six-day separations than when they have experienced only one.

And D. Vernon and his colleagues have also shown that, where children have had an unhappy experience in being separated, they are more likely to be upset by being admitted to hospital. But if children have been accustomed to separations that have not been upsetting, they may be less upset by hospital admission. This makes sense and suggests that it may be an advantage to accustom children to being with people other than their mothers.

The relationship with the mother before separation. As we have seen, the way in which a child responds to brief separations is not a simple index of the quality of his relationship with his mother. On the one hand, children seem more likely to protest their mother's departures if they have an intense and rewarding relationship with her; on the other, children with anxious or insecure relationships seem to be particularly disturbed by absence. Unfortunately we have very little evidence so far on how a child's relationship with his mother affects his response to longer separations. But the indications we have of children's emotional response to being admitted to hospital suggests that it does matter a great deal. Robert Hinde's studies of monkeys suggest that this may also be a key factor in the baby rhesus' reaction to longer separations. The baby monkeys who showed the greatest disturbance after the separation experience were those whose relationship with their mother before the separation was more difficult and "tense." Those whose attempts to achieve physical contact with their mothers had been more rejected, and had had to work hard to stay close, tended to be the most distressed during and after separation.

Also very important was the way the mother monkeys behaved when they were reunited with their babies. If the mother monkey had been removed to another pen while the baby remained in the home pen, she would herself be very disturbed by the removal. As she had to reestablish social relations with the other members of the group, she was much less able to cope with her baby, and less ready to respond to his demands. In these circumstances the baby monkey's distress was prolonged.

Obviously we would not want to draw a direct parallel here with the experiences of young children. But a useful point in thinking about human separations is that what disturbed the young monkeys was not so much the separation in itself but the disruption of the mother-child relationship and the mother's sense of ease in her environment.

Length of separation. We know very little about how the length of the separation affects the child's distress. Heinicke and Westheimer observed four children separated for seven to twenty-one weeks, and six separated for less than three weeks.[3] The children who were separated for the longer period showed more disturbance. And in the rhesus monkey studies, a thirteen-day separation caused greater distress than a six-day separation.

What are the long-term consequences for the child of these separation experiences that cause such distress at the time? One problem in assessing the results of studies of children who experience separation early in life is that for many children separation is combined with either very stressful or deprived conditions. Being separated from the home is associated with a host of other potentially upsetting experiences—going to the hospital, having a surgical operation, experiencing rather poor care in institutions, living in a relatively unfamiliar situation, and so on. It is also true that children who have to live in an institution or "strange place" for a time have often come from rather difficult home circumstances. All these experiences can add to the potentially disturbing effect of being separated from the family.

The general picture according to Michael Rutter, who has reviewed all the available evidence, is that short-term separations (not longer than a few nights) seem to have little effect on a child's intellectual or emotional behavior. There is a slightly increased risk of later psychological disturbance in the form of antisocial behavior, but in Rutter's own study, where the confusing effects of stress during separation were carefully distinguished, the results showed that separation is associated with antisocial behavior only where the separation is caused by family discord.[4] In these cases there is also likely to be some previous history of discord in the family.

A rather different emphasis, however, is given in a recent study of the long-term effects of hospital admissions by James Douglas. Douglas looked at the behavior in adolescence of a large number of children, all born in Great Britain during the same week.[5] The results showed that the children who had been admitted to hospital for more than one week, or admitted to hospital repeatedly, when younger than five years old were significantly more likely to show disturbed behavior as adolescents. They were more troublesome outside school, more likely to be delinquent, less likely to apply themselves in school (and in consequence more likely to be poor readers). They were also more likely to show unstable job patterns.

Of particular interest to us is the finding that the children who suffered most from early admission to hospital were those who were highly dependent on their mothers or who were under stress at the time of admission. If a child had just had a disturbing experience—a brother or sister had been born, or his mother had started work—then he was more likely to show disturbed behavior on being discharged from hospital, and also as an adolescent. If, however, his mother had been working for a time well before the hospital admission, he was less likely to be disturbed than the child of a nonworking mother.

Most studies have looked for unusual behavior in children, and they can give us no detailed picture of a child's behavior within what would be considered the normal range. It is possible, for example, that children who have experienced separation might be more apprehensive and upset by mildly stressful events than other children. A child's experiences may well color his response to difficult situations. There are clinical descriptions by James Robertson and John Bowlby that fit this picture. There are also interesting long-term observations of the rhesus monkeys who experienced separation. Within the family group their behavior was no different from that of other monkeys. But when tested in slightly strange situations at twelve and thirty months, they showed much more apprehension. They were less willing to approach a person offering food and tended to stay closer to the mother when moved to a strange cage. They also made shorter visits to a cage containing strange objects and were less active after having been frightened by some minor incident.

It is not possible, in the scope of this book, to discuss the effects of the deprivations children undergo in institutions and the problems of differentiating these from short- and long-term separation per se. A valuable overview can be found in Michael Rutter's *Maternal Deprivation Reassessed.*

WHAT CAUSES THE DISTRESS?

If we are trying to understand more clearly what is distressing about these long-term separation experiences, it can be very revealing to look at how the presence of others can relieve the distress.

Studies of children in nurseries and hospitals do show that the presence of familiar people other than the mother can greatly reduce distress. Heinecke and Westheimer, for instance, found that children who had a brother or sister with them in the nursery were much less distressed even when the sibling was only two or three and therefore much too young ever to have "mothered" the child in question or comforted him directly. From such observations it seems likely that how much comfort a person can provide during separation may depend on the nature of the child's prior relationship with him. It certainly does not depend simply on the amount of caregiving that person previously provided. Once again we note how important stimulating interaction—and not simply the relief of needs—can be in the formation of relationships. It is usually assumed by most researchers that the distress children show during a stay in hospital or institution is a product of their enforced separation from the mother. In fact, these experiences consist of separation from mother *and* father *and* siblings *and* home, as Rutter has pointed out.

Because the focus of research has been so much on the mother's relationship with the child, we know almost nothing, except at an anecdotal level, about children's reactions to being separated from their father or brothers and sisters. Heinecke's and Westheimer's evidence that the distress shown by children separated from home is greatly reduced by the presence of a sibling or a young friend raises a question of considerable importance. How far is the bond with the mother special and different in kind from the child's relationships with other people? Bowlby argues that the first attachment a child forms is different in kind from the relationships he forms with other familiar people, and that children have a built-in tendency to form this special attachment to one person. But if the most crucial aspects of this attachment are that it provides security and comfort, and if these distress-reducing aspects are also present in the child's relationship with his brothers and sisters, father, grandmother, and so on, then this must cast doubt on the special nature of the child's bond to the mother. The idea that the child is born with an urge to form a bond with one person is also difficult to reconcile with the evidence that young children may become attached to several people. It seems much more likely that the numbers of people to whom a child develops attachments depends on his social and family setting, and on how rich and varied it is.

Looking at what modifies the traumatic effects of longer separation has helped our understanding of what causes the distress in a number of ways. (These points will be very important when we come to assess John Bowlby's concept of attachment.) First, though it does seem that the distress is due to the child's sense of loss of the loved one, we don't really know how far it may be due to the loss of other attachments, or even to the lack of opportunity to develop a new attachment. This point is illustrated by the moving films of children's responses to separation experiences made by James and Joyce Robertson. The Robertsons studied the responses to separation of four children whose mothers went to hospital by themselves combining the roles of foster parents and observers and bringing the children into their own home for the course of the separation.[6] They compared the reaction of these children with the reaction of children who were placed in residential institutions while their mothers were away. The "fostered" children, who each received the individual care of Mrs. Robertson, did show some signs of insecurity but no signs of distress on the scale of those children who were left in residential care. How did the experiences of the four children looked after by the Robertsons differ? Three points should be noted. First, they received "mothering" from one individual—very different from the multiple caregivers they would have had in an institution. Moreover, the Robertsons followed the children's known daily routine and the childrearing pattern to which they were used. They gave each child intense and continuing friendship. Second, each child had met the Robertsons before the separation, and this brief familiarization may have helped to provide comfort. Third, the Robertsons talked to the children about their mothers and tried to keep their memories of the mothers alive; regular visits were paid by the fathers during the mothers' absence.

In comparing the relative ease with which the four children

coped with the separation experience, and the desperate distress of the children who were in institutions for equivalent periods, we are not in a position to distinguish clearly how far success was due to the fact that the children could and did develop attachments to the Robertsons, or to the fact that the children's relationships with their mother was "supported" by continued discussion and reference, or to the familiarity with the Robertsons themselves.

The second point to be emphasized is that it is not necessarily separation from the mother exclusively that seems to be the crucial factor. How much it *is* the mother's absence that matters will depend on the quality of the child's relationship with her, on the breadth and depth of his other attachments, and of course on whether other family members also disappear completely from the child's experience during the course of the separation.

The third point is that we simply do not have enough systematic information to know how important separation from the home environment is in causing distress. There are few observations of children left at home while their mothers are absent, and even in these few cases other familiar people have continued to be present in the home. It seems very likely that both familiar people and setting are helpful in lessening the distress.

What can we learn from these studies about the ways in which young children form relationships? The evidence that young brothers and sisters and friends can and do provide comfort is further evidence that it is exciting interaction that is crucial. This change of emphasis in what we see as important in the growth of relationships has meant that research attention is now focused on reciprocal interaction, on *mutual* gazing and timing of movements.

SECURITY, COMFORT, AND THE DEVELOPMENT OF SOCIAL RELATIONSHIPS

There is, then, considerable doubt about how exclusively comfort and security are bound up with the main "attachment figure." What connection is there between these security aspects of the child's first attachments and the way in which his other social relationships develop?

Bowlby uses the experiments of Harlow with rhesus babies to illustrate how important physical contact with the mother figure is for the development of security, and how important this security is for the development of the ability to cope and for the development of social behavior both with friends of the child's own age and with other adults. Harlow sees the stage of physical contact and comfort as vital in the development of social behavior. "Intimate physical contact is the variable of primary importance in enabling the infant to pass from the stage of comfort and attachment to the state of security, specific security to a specific mother figure."

But a very different view of the importance of the comfort and security aspects of attachment is put forward by Lawrence Kohlberg.[7] He sees the security side of the relationship as less important and essentially irrelevant to the development of true social behavior. For Kohlberg the most important features of human social attachments are those of sharing, communication, and cooperation "between selves recognizing each other as selves." He agrees that the baby's positive attachments grow out of his natural desire to take part in social exchange, but believes that the contact and security Bowlby emphasizes play little if any part in the development of true social interaction. He also cites Harlow's experiments with surrogate mothers, pointing out that while the cloth mother did provide a safe base from which to explore, and provided comfort in a fear-invoking situation, these monkeys did not go on to cope adequately as adults with social situations. Another group of baby rhesus, who were reared solely with other baby monkeys, did grow up to perform adequately, both sexually and as parents. It is the experience of reciprocal play with others of the same age, Kohlberg argues, that forms a base for the development of complementary sharing behavior. Needing someone for comfort and physical security does not in itself develop social behavior, because the baby has no motive to interact with, or be guided by, his source of security. Further, it is doubtful whether the relationship with the mother is more important than the relationship with brothers or sisters in the development of social behavior.

What Kohlberg has underlined for us is the importance of play with others. It does not necessarily follow that it must be play with children of the same age. For many children (and indeed for some nonhuman primates, such as chimpanzees) early play is largely play with the mother. The fact that in many families it is the mother who both provides physical comfort and security *and* is the chief playmate may in itself have consequences for a child's emotional and social development. It is ironic that, since Kohlberg put forward these ideas, there has been a great deal of work on the earliest stages of reciprocal interaction—but *all* of it has been done by looking at the mother with the baby. We still have no knowledge at all about how much of this reciprocal play goes on with other members of the family or about how it differs in quality with different members of the family.

These disagreements make clear how little we yet know about the links between the physical contact and security aspects of relationships and other aspects of social behavior. We would probably expect an eighteen-month-old child who fell over and hurt himself when playing with his friends to go to his mother for comfort, but to be eager to go back and spend time with his friends as soon as he cheered up. But we know so little, in a systematic way, about the ordinary communication between young children in a family that we might be wrong in assuming that children would always prefer to seek physical comfort and security from their mothers. Should we assume, as Eleanor Maccoby and John Masters do, that the baby's simple attachment to one figure becomes differentiated by the age of three or four into "proximity-seeking" and "attention-seeking," two forms of behavior directed at different types of people?[8] They suggest that the people these different sorts of behavior are directed to will be determined by the sort of response the people give. Adults will be more likely to respond satisfactorily to the child's wish for physical contact and comfort while other children may be just as stimulating to interact with. When we draw up such schemes for the development of "systems" of behavior, we may be in danger of mistaking what is in fact a typically Western pattern of family life for something universally true of humans. Rudolph Schaffer and Peggy Emerson presented evidence that the number and breadth of the attachments that a one-year-old developed were a reflection of the social setting in which he was raised. If we look at some recent studies of children raised in group care, we can see that our views on the mother as the source of security and physical comfort may well reflect our own experience of the nuclear family rather than a biologically established pattern.

DAY CARE

There have now been a number of studies made of the effects of day care on children's early relationships. None of the studies of groups where the children had started to attend the day-care center before the age of one showed any difference in the patterns of attachment between each child and his mother. However, one follow-up study of such a group has some interesting implications for our ideas on attachment. Here, children from one day-care center were observed when they started nursery schools at the age of two and three. The children in this center had been kept in small groups of three or four from the time that they entered—the average age was nine months—until they went on to nursery school. When these children first entered nursery school they were found to differ in their behavior from the family-reared children. First they adjusted to the new environment much more easily: in the first week they showed less tension, interacted more with other children, and were happier. They were observed again after four months and after seven months in the nursery, and were found to be less cooperative and amenable to the teacher's wishes than the family-reared children. The impression one gets is that the young children who had been "brought up" together from their first year are very close to each other; they derive considerable security from each other's presence, which helps them to cope with and enjoy the new nursery environment. We have descriptions of the close ties between children reared in kibbutzim that parallel these findings in interesting ways.

These results show once again how ignorant we are about the flexibility and the complexity of early relationships. We are particularly ignorant about children's relationships with other children—recall the studies of babies' reactions to strangers, where the child stranger, unlike the adult, was greeted with delight. A child may have relationships with his mother, father, grandmother and grandfather, brothers and sisters, and neighbors and other children. Each of these relationships may be rather different and may be differently influenced by different situations. We need to know a great deal more about this range of relationships before we can say that each child has *one* original attachment or that later relationships develop and can only develop from this base.

PHYSICAL CONTACT AND SECURITY

We also do not have a very clear picture of what developments take place in the way a young child seeks physical comfort and security when distressed. By the age of three or four there is certainly a fall-off in the child's eagerness to be near his mother, even in new situations, but whether the original desire for physical contact is replaced by other forms of attention seeking is much less certain. As the child becomes older he becomes more involved with other people, more mobile, and more competent at maintaining contact with those he loves by talking to them and showing them things. In general terms, the early forms of maintaining contact with the mother, by touching and keeping close, change to forms of maintaining contact over a distance, by looking and talking. But there is no simple pattern of development here; the one-year-old who stays close to mother is not necessarily going to be a three-year-old who constantly looks at and talks to her parents.

Quite a lot of research has been done on "dependent" behavior in three- and four-year-olds—their asking for attention and help and their wanting to be near adults, for example. But much of this research is confusing, and it certainly does not tell a neat or simple story. For example, one study of nursery-school children found that the girls who wanted to be physically close to the teacher were also the most likely to want other forms of comfort, reassurance, and attention, and that they also demanded a good deal of attention from their mothers. But the boys who wanted physical comfort and closeness to the teacher did not necessarily seem to want other sorts of attention from their mothers. In another study those children rated by the teacher as wanting a lot of physical closeness were also likely to be rated as seeking a lot of attention generally. However, there was no relation between these measures of the children's behavior and how upset they were likely to be on being separated from their mothers.

These results are confusing if we try to fit them into a single system of children's dependent behavior; and the same sort of confusion will probably arise if we try to see later behavior as growing from a single, simple attachment system in the child's first nineteen months or so. One way of learning more about the possible range of children's relationships is to look at studies of children in other cultures, and it is to these we turn next.

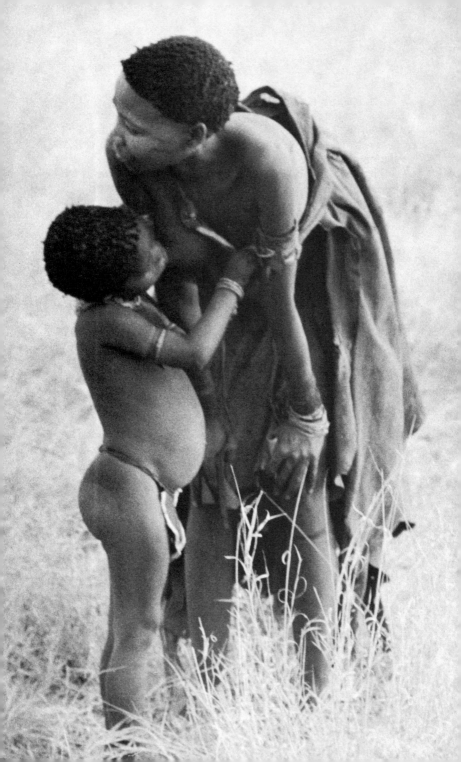

8 / Other Cultures

In Britain or America, when a baby begins to fret he may well be left to cry for a long time before he gets any attention or before he stops from sheer exhaustion. This may be because he is alone in a room and no one hears him, or it may be because on principle he is left to cry it out. As we have seen, psychologists disagree widely about the consequences of this experience, repeated as it may be many hundreds of times. Many feel that such experiences play an important part in leading to a difficult and ambivalent relationship between mother and child. They consider that a quick and sensitive response to distress is the natural way for a mother to respond, a way that has become overridden in our modern technological world by anxieties about spoiling and by a preoccupation with the importance of the child's independence. In many less "developed" societies, by contrast, the babies are never left to cry but are responded to immediately when they fret. The baby of a !Kung bushman in the Kalahari, for example, is carried on his mother's back for most of the day, in contact with his mother's warm skin; he is put to the breast well before he reaches the point of fretting, and he is played with and handled constantly by loving friendly people.[1] The striking differences in the early experience of comfort and distress between our own culture and that of the bushmen is certainly of enormous interest, but we need to think very carefully about exactly what we can learn from these differences.

Descriptions from ethnographic studies are bound to raise the question: What are the consequences of intense and constant contact with a responsive mother? In themselves, however, such descriptions cannot provide us with the answer. Although we

87

have many fascinating descriptions from anthropologists of the diverse ways in which babies are cared for and loved in different societies, the societies they describe differ in so many other ways that it would be impossible definitely to link the early childrearing practices to any broad differences in later personality or in social relationships. This does not mean that no one has attempted to draw conclusions of this kind. In fact, many of the earlier descriptions of childrearing patterns jump happily from accounts of comforting, feeding, or weaning to broad pronouncements about the personality or temperament of the adult group.

Margaret Mead, for instance, in *Sex and Temperament in Three Primitive Societies* gives us a vivid description of the differences in temperament and behavior of two New Guinea societies, the mountain-dwelling Arapesh and the river-dwelling Mundugumor, in which the early experiences of the children are presented as an important source of later personality differences. The Arapesh she characterizes as people with easy, gentle, receptive personalities, with both males and females having a warm and maternal temperament. During the first months of life, the Arapesh baby is never far from someone's arms; he is suckled whenever he cries and held a great deal. "A child's crying is a tragedy to be avoided at any cost." Arapesh children develop a wide circle of people they can trust—people who fill their early months with love.

In contrast to the Arapesh, for whom "growing food and children is the greatest adventure of their lives," the Mundugumor society is marked by ruthless individualism, aggression, and competitive enmity. Almost from birth, the Mundugumor baby is kept in a stiff carrying basket, too thick for body contact with his caregiver and too big for him to see out of. When he cries, he is seldom fed at once. The standard method of soothing a fretful infant is for some bystander to scratch the outside of the basket, making a harsh sound. If the baby does not stop crying he is eventually suckled, but during the feed there is none of the dallying pleasure enjoyed by the Arapesh mother and baby. The baby is fed as quickly as possible, held in a standing position. The child develops a fighting technique of feeding, sucking very vigorously and frequently choking; this angers the mother and infuriates the baby, and feeds become periods of anger and struggle. The breast is only given to the older crawling babies when they are really thought to be hungry, never to comfort a baby who is frightened or in pain. Weaning too is a hostile process; while a Mundugumor child will continue to try to reach his mother's breasts, he avoids other contact with her; he never attempts to lie in her lap "unless so ill that he is almost unconscious of what he does."

Margaret Mead shows that the differences in childrearing are typical of the broad differences between the two societies. What we do not know is how far the actual practices of comforting and attentiveness shown by the Arapesh are in themselves important in the development of the warm receptive personalities of the Arapesh; many of the two societies' later socialization practices and cultural patterns differ, and these may well be equally (if not more) important. Little effort is made to distinguish systematically between cause and consequence in the account of Arapesh childrearing and personality patterns. If we are to begin to understand the importance of the widely different experiences of early comfort and distress undergone by babies in different cultures, we need to have very precise and systematic information about the details of the early experience, and about the later differences in personality and relationships, and we also need to know a great deal about other aspects of the society. Since we are only just beginning to understand what a complicated business it is to trace the origins of individual differences in our own culture, the leap to pronouncing so boldly on what is important in other cultures seems rash.

There are a few studies that provide information systematic enough for us to begin to grasp the origins of differences between young children in different cultures, even if we cannot extrapolate from these to differences in adult personality. One detailed study, by William Caudill and Helen Weinstein, comparing Japanese and American middle-class mothers and babies, showed pronounced differences between the cultures in the care of three-month-old babies.[2] The American mothers had a stimulating and lively approach to their babies, moving them about vigorously, looking at and chatting to them. The Japanese mothers had a much gentler, soothing approach, spending more time quieting, lulling, and rocking their babies. A further major difference between the cultures was found in the *links* between the behavior of baby and mother: the American mother responded to happy noises from the baby by stimulating him further with talking and playing. The Japanese mother interacted more with her baby to soothe him when he was fretful, and did not respond to or build up on his happy vocal behavior in the same way. Parallel to these findings there were marked differences between the babies in the two cultures, with the American babies being more active, more happily vocal, and more exploratory than the quieter and more passive Japanese babies.

If we suppose that, as well as differences in caregiving styles, there are differences in the characteristics of the babies themselves in these two groups, the problems of untangling the origins of any single difference are considerable. Caudill and Weinstein consider that the differences in the caregiving styles between the American and Japanese mothers are so great that one can reasonably attribute differences in the babies at three months entirely to cultural differences in caregiving. But it is possible that the babies in the two groups were different from their earliest days; as we noted in Chapter Two, wide cross-cultural differences have been shown in studies of newborn babies, and differences in response to soothing and in abilities of self-quieting were particularly marked. These differences may very well influence the way a mother behaves with her baby. This means that to understand fully the origins of the cross-cultural differences at three months, either in the mothers' style or in the babies' behavior, we would need to trace the development of both from the earliest days.

Even though our systematic information is often scanty, we do of course know enough to have some broad sense of which factors are likely to be important. The descriptions of other cultures are tantalizing—suggestive and provocative but never quite definitive. In her striking account of an Indonesian people, the people of Alor, Cora Du Bois describes how the mother, two weeks after giving birth, returns to the fields to work without taking the new baby with her.[3] He is left for the whole day at home in the care of father, older sibling, or grandmother. This practice results in great variation in the amount of attention and feeding that babies get over the first year. Every child is nursed by other adult women, at one time or another, but these substitutes are no more consistently available than the mother herself.

The baby is not left alone, even when asleep, and he is not left to cry, but since the breast can rarely be given to comfort, a variety of other soothing techniques are used. One of the favorites is to massage the genitals gently—a method used particularly by the child caregivers.

Such descriptions give us intriguing glimpses of other worlds; but they can do more. In particular they can alert us to the danger of extrapolating too generally from our own culture. The study of the people of Alor shows that it is not always the mother who provides comfort and care in the early weeks. What will these differences mean for the children's developing relationships? We are in no position to give definite answers to such questions, though Du Bois notes that the child's dependence on his mother is much less marked than in our own society and that the children have warm relationships with many other people of different ages.

But descriptions of preagricultural hunter-gatherer societies, in particular, have been used in a much more definite way to throw light on human development. It has been argued that, since man has lived as a hunter-gatherer for more than 99 percent of the three million years he has existed, we may learn a great deal about what lies beneath most human behavior from studying people living this kind of life today. Distinctively human patterns of affection and emotion and of social relationships, it is claimed, have evolved in the context of a hunter-gatherer existence. More specifically it has been proposed that, by looking at the way babies are cared for and loved in societies living in ecological and social conditions that closely resemble the conditions in which man evolved, we can learn more about the "natural" relationship between mother and baby. Descriptions of hunter-gatherer societies such as the !Kung stress the continual contact between mother and baby, the responsiveness of the mother to her baby's distress, and the absolute indulgence shown toward his dependent behavior. Study of the !Kung showed, for example, that during the first year the average amount of time that elapsed between a baby's fretting and his mother's responding was six seconds. The argument about what we can learn from such patterns is sometimes presented as an extension of the discussion about what we can learn from studying nonhuman primates: if we go against the "natural" biological predispositions suggested by the evidence from nonhuman primates and hunter-gatherer societies, we run the risk of distorting the child's development. This argument centers particularly on comfort and distress because it is here that the differences between the hunter-gatherer societies and our own are so extreme. Indeed the picture of !Kung infancy has been taken as providing powerful evidence for John Bowlby's theory of attachment. The babies in !Kung society certainly develop very intense attachments to their mothers.

But there are two important points to make here. First, can we really learn much about man's biological adaptation from looking at present-day hunter-gatherer societies? They have, after all, like all human societies had several million years to evolve, and we are on shaky ground if we conclude that the !Kung are representative of early men. We do not know enough of the range of conditions under which hunter-gatherer societies evolved, or of the consequent range of variation between these societies, to put so much weight on this particular group. Why should we assume that the Kalahari !Kung patterns are the natural ones we are biologically adapted to?

Second, even if our knowledge of man's prehistory were more firmly based, would this help us to look after babies in our own culture? We cannot know what is natural, and even if we could, we would not necessarily know that it would be a good thing to recommend it. Patterns of social behavior, even with young babies, are part of a culture, and the idea that there is a biological pattern of relationships divorced from culture is misleading. We are very far from understanding in what sense social behavior is constrained or influenced by biological adaptations, or from understanding the relationship between social behavior and genetics. The fact that man, who evolved in a hunter-gatherer environment, has so rapidly developed such an astonishing variety of social patterns in other cultural environments might be taken as an argument against biological adaptation to a hunter-gatherer existence as crucial to human social development.

Further, we do not know what the consequences would be if we were to recommend that mothers followed a particular type of caregiving borrowed from another culture: we have to take account of the culture for which that infant is being prepared. If we did try to bring our babies up in a manner resembling the !Kung hunter-gatherers, with constant physical contact and immediate attention, our lives as parents who must function in an industrial society, without the supporting group that !Kung parents have, might be intolerably difficult. !Kung parents apparently have a great deal of leisure time, and probably spend more time than Western parents sitting around in groups and chatting. Children brought up in this way might well find it difficult, too, to adjust to life in the world outside the family, which after all does not closely resemble the !Kung Kalahari life.

Sometimes, of course, our biological knowledge can help us to understand how modern practices that "override" biology have altered behavior, but these instances are likely to be rather small-scale examples. Take, for example, our finding that breastfed babies in the Cambridge study awoke and cried much more frequently than bottle-fed babies in the first ten days after birth, becoming restless and crying within two to three hours after the previous feeding. This frequent waking and crying had a dramatic effect on the numbers of women who continued to breastfeed, for many felt that the normal baby who was getting enough milk would be sleeping for four hours between feeds. Now if we look at the composition of the milks of various mammals, we find that there is a relationship between the protein content of the milk and the frequency of feeds that the mother gives the infant; this relationship cuts across the different groups of mammals. If we arrange the milks of the various mammals in order according to the protein content of the milk, and the frequency of the feeds, we find that human breast milk with its comparatively low protein content puts us among the species who need to be "continuously" fed. Bottle milk, on the other hand, with its higher protein content, is comparable to the milks of species that feed less frequently. It is understandable, then, that the breastfed babies, at least in the early days of lactation, demand frequent feeds. By introducing bottle milk, we have altered the "natural" pattern of feeding contact between mother and baby. Of course this new understanding of the basis of the different patterns of demand from the babies does not tell us what the implications of the different patterns of contact are for the developing relationship between mother and baby. The biological basis of the attachment between mother and baby is so little understood at present that we are not in a position to judge whether this sort of change in contact patterns is disadvantageous for the child's emotional development.

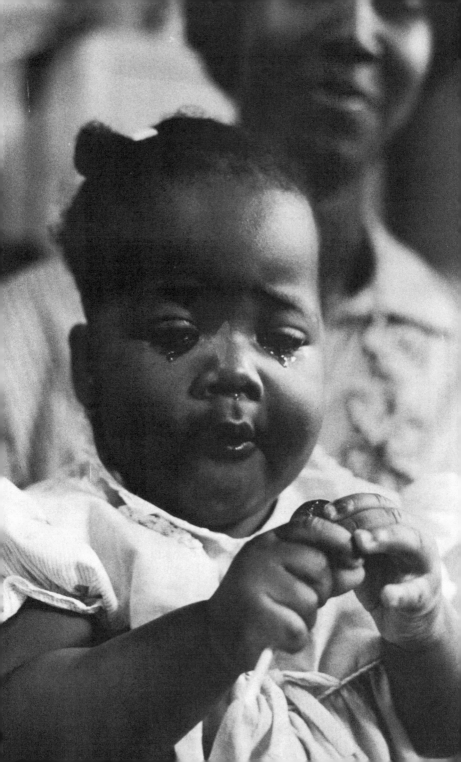

9 / The Development of Understanding

We have already touched on the role of the early relationship between mother and child in the development of communication, understanding, and language. The child's experience of distress and his mother's part in relieving that distress and maintaining his sense of security play a central part in our ideas about this issue. We look next at some of these ideas and at the studies carried out to test them. How is the baby's physical and emotional state related to advances in his behavior? Does he learn new things when he is calm and happy, or when he is in a state of tension and need? How does the mother's loving involvement influence the baby's progress through the developmental changes of the first two years?

THE STATE OF THE BABY AND HIS INTELLECTUAL DEVELOPMENT

If you try to make a very young baby follow an object with his eyes, holding it in front of him and moving it to and fro, you will find that your success at catching his attention will depend largely on how calm and alert he is. If he is very irritable and on edge he will probably not attend at all. If he is just a little fretful he may calm down and watch with interest, ceasing to move and fuss. If he is in a calm and wakeful state he will watch and follow keenly. The fact that babies do attend much more in an alert and inactive state implies that they are much more likely to learn about the world around them and to adapt their behavior to new circumstances in the way that is so important in development.

Peter Wolff showed, as we have seen, that by giving a baby

95

interesting objects to look at, he could keep the baby quiet and attentive when otherwise he would be dozing off or fussing. As the baby grows up, not only does he get better at voluntarily keeping himself looking at things that interest him or away from things that don't, but the range of events that have "meaning" and interest for him increases. He knows that his father's entrance heralds a game, that his mother's preparations mean a bottle is coming. He also develops new ways of finding out about physical objects. It looks as if the child's periods of alertness increase at points where the child acquires new physical skills and hence new ways of exploring the world—the range of things he can investigate increases, for instance, when he begins to coordinate hand and eye. It seems that the baby first manages these longer periods of alertness after he has been fed and changed —that is, after his mother has removed sources of distress. This plausibly suggests that the best state in which the baby makes new discoveries about what he can do, or about what the world is like, is when he is calm and alert, not when he is bothered by pain or hunger. According to this picture, then, the mother's ability to keep the baby calm and happy is a key factor in providing him with the best circumstances for learning. Some observations by Anneliese Korner and Rose Grobstein illustrate this well.[1] They found that when crying babies are picked up and held to the shoulder, they not only quiet down but also become alert and scan the environment. So they systematically compared the babies' reactions to different sorts of mothering actions. They tried putting the baby on either shoulder, or just sitting him up so that he was vertical but not cuddled. They found that handling alone did not induce alertness but that holding the baby to the shoulder was very effective. The mother's usual response—picking up the baby—will thus provide the best encouragement for his attending to the world around him and of course for learning about her.

Some of the most recent work on the exchange between mothers and infants has taken the form of detailed analysis of films and videotapes of mothers and babies playing and "talking" together. One of the striking features of this interaction turns out to be the way a mother subtly and sensitively modifies and times her interventions and exchanges with the baby to keep him happy and alert. Films by Colwyn Trevarthen have shown that the "communicative ability" of the babies in these interchanges is far more complex than their other abilities; Trevarthen has gone on to emphasize just how important for the development of human intelligence this exchange between baby and adult must be.

Trevarthen's observations, and those of Korner and Grobstein, fit well with the notion of the emotional shelter that the mother provides and that enables the baby to turn outward from absorption in himself. But, as noted earlier, other psychologists have taken a very different view of the relation between the child's emotional states and advances in intellectual behavior. Freud and René Spitz, for example, both stressed the great influence of frustration on learning. The opposite emphases stem from a difference in the central concerns of psychoanalysts on the one hand and of developmental psychologists on the other. The psychoanalysts are interested in what drives a child to *try*, and it is clear that frustration is important here. But most psychologists have been primarily interested in what enhances the capacity of the child to *succeed* in learning. This distinction has profound implications. In stressful frustrating circumstances, though the urgency of the child's need will make him form some concepts, they may not necessarily be the most appropriate ones. The development of fantasy does not necessarily help the development of rational understanding. As for the question of the circumstances in which children learn, it certainly seems plausible that a child can learn under mildly frustrating circumstances. Franz Plooij has observed that young chimps living in the wild do learn some food-finding skills such as termite digging at the point when the mother chimpanzee stops sharing her own food with them. In this situation frustration and hunger drives the young chimps to try for themselves. It is possible that other sorts of frustration might push children into learning. But descriptions of how disorganized and chaotic behavior becomes when a baby is in extreme states of distress tend to suggest that these are *not* the circumstances that help him to make discoveries about the world.

Although psychoanalytic theory assumes that emotional tension plays a crucial part in influencing the child's thought and action, Piaget's theory of intellectual development—the most comprehensive scheme that we have—does not give the child's emotional state an important place. Piaget noted that fluctuations in the child's emotional state could affect the child's maturity of behavior, but most of his writing implies that he did not feel this had any important bearing on the child's comprehension of the world. His theory, for example, attributes no importance to the pleasure involved in exchanges with parents. When Piaget made observations of his own children, he selected those periods when the child was performing at his best without, for the most part, noting his emotional state. However, he did suggest that when a young baby is in a state of mild tension, such as slight hunger, his coordination might be improved. There may well be changes with age in the way tension affects the baby's coordination and behavior—it is an area we know very little about.

One of the problems we face in investigating this issue of when the child is making advances in behavior is that it is difficult to know on what occasions a child is learning something genuinely new, or is developing a new way of coping with a problem. We cannot assume, simply because a three-month-old baby is looking attentively at a colored rattle, or an eighteen-month-old is playing with sand and water, that either child is learning anything. And so even if we say that a child is more likely to play with sand and water when he is in a certain emotional state, we cannot necessarily pin down the points at which, in his play, he is making new discoveries. We must pay attention to an event in the outside world to understand it, but it would be absurd to assume that this is enough on its own. One way of trying to get around the problem is to watch a child so frequently, and for such long periods, that one gets some idea of his particular level of understanding and can note when more advanced patterns of behavior first appear. And this general approach was exactly the one that Piaget used in observing his own children. It has also been used by Sibylle Escalona in an investigation of children during their first eight months.[2] An examination of her findings brings us to the issue of how a child's interaction with an adult influences the advances he makes in developing his skills.

INTERACTION WITH ADULTS AND THE DEVELOPMENT OF INTELLECTUAL SKILLS

Parents support and encourage their children's intellectual development in a number of different ways. We have seen that from his earliest days a child begins to take part in communication through interaction with his mother. We have seen how important the early exchange between mother and baby is: in the early months the mother supports and extends the baby's interest in the exchange most effectively; her loving attention to his needs and her interpretation of his wishes form the basis for real communication of shared meanings.

We have also discussed at some length the difference that his mother's presence makes to the way a child explores a new environment and investigates what is unfamiliar. In a very general sense, then, she plays a crucial role in enabling the child to learn about the world. Escalona's observations give us some specific examples of the context in which particular skills first appear.

She noted that a baby often first displayed some new awareness or skill when happily playing games with his mother—the discovery of the delights of banging bricks together, for example—but that these new skills usually seemed to be a passive response, with his mother leading the game. It was when the child was playing alone with toys or objects that he first actively used these new skills, as he explored and exploited the properties of his toys. According to Escalona, it was only after mastering his skill with objects that he began to use his new ability in exchanges with other people. But interaction with the mother did not affect all children in the same way: a mother's active play had a greater impact on the level of maturity of the child's play if he was a placid baby rather than an active one. This finding parallels Schaffer's findings that long periods in hospital (where babies naturally get less attention than they would at home) are more likely to hold back the development of the inactive than the active babies.

These observations do not suggest that the children showed more mature behavior when they were in a state of frustration or distress. And in fact a study by David Wood, Jerome Bruner, and Gail Ross of the way mothers tutor children and encourage new skills shows that an important feature of this tutoring is that the mother manages to keep the child happy and at a high peak of interest.[3] Secure and happy play periods in which the child can practice and develops new abilities do seem to be very important. Bruner points out that, if we compare different species of primates, we find that in the more highly evolved species like chimpanzees the young spend more time playing. He links this opportunity for play with the development of tool using and communications and emphasizes that it is particularly in the context of secure and close interaction with their mothers that primates develop skills.

For the development of language, the secure and comfortable daily exchange between the child and an adult familiar with his interests is certainly important. When we look carefully at the situations in which babies take the first steps toward using language—understanding and taking part in exchanges that lead to the first words—we find that it is the interchange between adult and baby in tension-free play and easy-going routine that matters a great deal.

Thus the mother's role in the child's intellectual development is important at a number of different levels: in the early sequences of interaction where the child's level of excitement is carefully monitored and controlled by his parent; in the later interaction sequences when he develops a sense of the social meaning of actions and objects; in introducing new skills in playful exchanges; and in providing general security enabling the child to explore the world. Still another way in which the mother's behavior has been linked to the child's intellectual development has to do with his sense of mastery and competence: the mother's response to his distress in the early months is seen as first giving him a sense of control and efficacy—making him feel that his environment can be affected, and by him.

The observations discussed so far have all concerned the importance for the developing child of these very general aspects of maternal comfort. But it has also been suggested that differences between mothers in their particular responses to distress can lead to differences between individual babies in intellectual development. A number of studies seem to support the idea that children whose mothers have been very responsive to their signals are developmentally more advanced. What particular aspects of responsiveness are the ones that matter? In what way could they be affecting the child's intellectual development?

In one study of five-month-old babies, Leon Yarrow and his colleagues found that the babies whose mothers had responded quickly and consistently to distress scored highly on mental tests, particularly on those tests involving the babies' interest and persistence in playing with objects. They were persistent in reaching for objects, more interested in manipulating new objects, and explored them with greater attention. Yarrow concluded that the interest and drive of these babies had been fostered by mothers who, by responding quickly to the babies' distress signals, had helped them to develop a sense that they could influence and control their own environment. He thought that mothers' responses to crying not only explained the development of the children's general sense of efficacy but also influenced strongly how motivated each of them was to explore and master his environment.

Yarrow's notions were supported by the results of another study. Clarke-Stewart looked at how various different aspects of maternal care and responsiveness affected a child's intellectual development later on, in the second year of life.[4] She found that the mothers who were most promptly responsive to the babies' smiles, looks, and noises at eleven months had children who several months later were the most intellectually advanced. The verbal and social stimulation, the amount of positive emotion the mother showed toward the child, and the amount of time she spent playing with him all contributed positively to his intellectual development. However, the mother's response to the baby's distress did *not* follow this pattern. That was found to be related not to the child's intellectual development, but rather to the quality of the physical attachment he showed for his mother. For the sorts of intellectual development taking place in the second year of the child's life, then, it seems that the mother's response to the child's looks, smiles, and "talking" may be very important, but that her response to the child's distress has more important effects on his emotional development.

In a third study Sylvia Bell explored the consequences of individual differences in mothers' responsiveness and sensitivity for one particular aspect of intellectual development: object permanence.[5] Piaget had hypothesized that babies develop a sense that people continue to exist when out of sight before they develop an equivalent awareness that objects are permanent. He thought this would happen because people are so much more interesting to a baby, because the mother is such a constant feature of the baby's world, and because she continually comes and goes in a way often directly related to his signals. If Piaget were right, it would follow that a nine-month-old would be capable of playing hide-and-seek with his mother, but would not search for an object beneath a cloth; he would not realize it still existed even if it were hidden as he watched. In Bell's study, most of the babies did develop a sense of their mother's permanence before they developed an awareness of the permanence of objects. She found that the few (seven) babies for whom this symbolic sense developed first with objects, and only later with people, had relationships with their mothers of a different quality from the majority. Following a brief separation from their mothers in a laboratory, they were much less likely to rush up for cuddling, as most would. They were either ambivalent toward the mother's return or were more interested in the toys in the room.

Bell interpreted these results as showing that a child needs a harmonious relationship with his mother to develop a sense of her permanence first. She felt, too, that the other course of development, the sense of object permanence first, was atypical since it was less common and since these children tended to be relatively slow in their later development of a sense of person permanence. Since Mary Ainsworth's studies had linked the child's ambivalent reaction to the way his mother responded to his distress, Bell felt she had demonstrated that the emotional quality of the relationship between mother and child was one of the crucial factors influencing intellectual development—at least at this important stage. This interesting study is now being repeated with a larger sample, which is important because we need to know more about the individual differences between the children. There seem to be two rather different patterns of behavior among the seven babies who developed object permanence first. Four of them were more interested in objects than in their mother's return after separation; the other three were definitely ambivalent and upset in their reaction to their mother's return. It is important to distinguish these two types of response if we are to understand how differences in mothering style have influenced the course of development.

THE LONG-TERM SIGNIFICANCE OF MOTHERING STYLES

If we have demonstrated a link between the parents' caregiving style and their baby's intellectual development during the first eighteen months or so of his life, what can this tell us about

the baby's future development? It has become a cliché to emphasize the importance of the earliest experiences on young children,
but we need to think more carefully about the evidence on which
this idea is based. This is particularly true for intellectual development. It is notoriously difficult to link intellectual differences
in development during the first two years with individual differences in intellectual development later on. Children who score
highly in intelligence tests when they are two or more continue
to do relatively well in these tests. But no one has shown a connection between scoring highly on the various tests developed to
assess infant intelligence below two and doing well on later tests
of ability, beyond a continuity (for girls only) in some aspects of
verbal skill.

This discontinuity between "baby intelligence" and later intelligence can be interpreted in two ways. It could be that we are
not measuring the appropriate aspects of young children's development and abilities when they are very small, and that this is
why we have failed to show a connection with later individual
differences. Or it could be that there is a real discontinuity here,
and that the sorts of development in intellectual capacity that
take place after the child is talking are unrelated to what has
been happening over the first two years. If that is true, then the
sorts of experience that influence a child's early progress may
well not be relevant in any systematic way to his later intellectual development. The importance of a mother's response to her
child's distress would in that case have to be reconsidered. We
would have to ask what connection there was either between a
mother's response to distress in the first year and later intellectual development or between the mother's response to distress in
the first year and those aspects of *her own* later behavior which
do influence the child's development.

Some findings from our Cambridge study are relevant here.[6]
We looked at the mothers' interest in and responsiveness to their
babies over the first fourteen months. We also took measures of
each child's intellectual ability later, including his IQ at four and
a half years. We noted that, although mothers were not consistently different from one another in how they responded to their
babies' crying over the first year, they *were* in their interest in
talking to their babies, in engaging them in play with objects,
and in responding to the babies' noises. Further, these individual
differences in the mothers' behavior were found to be related to

the babies' interest in talking to their mothers, in showing and giving them things. Now it is just these aspects of exchange and communication between mother and child at fourteen months that we might assume to be good predictors of later intellectual development. However, when we looked at the way the children in the sample performed in the IQ test at four and a half, we found no connection at all. Yet there *was* a link between the later IQ and another measure of the mother's behavior at fourteen months: a measure not of *whether* the mother replied to the child's noises (as the responsiveness measures had been) but of *how* she replied to him. We found, in fact, that the children who did well on IQ tests at four and a half years had mothers who when talking to their children at fourteen months had been particularly accepting in their verbal response to the child's words and actions. These mothers frequently replied in a way that showed approval, agreement, or acceptance ("Good—yes, that's the way," or "It's a dog, yes").

What these findings showed, then, was that a particular style of response and interest in the child during the first year was not directly related to those aspects of intelligence that are measured in tests later on. A particular kind of verbal response from the mother when the child was fourteen months did relate to later IQ. Incidentally this study provided another example of the danger of assuming that a measure of the mother's responsiveness is independent of the characteristics of the child. We found that the responsiveness of the mother depended on how many of the baby's noises were demands for objects and requests for help.

One possible reason why continuities from the first year on are not easy to find could be that both mothers and (perhaps even more) fathers may change in their interest and feelings toward their babies as they grow up. A parent who is really not deeply involved with a five-month-old may become much more drawn to a talkative two-year-old.

It seems rather doubtful then that we will find simple connections between individual differences in the ability of five-month-old babies and the abilities of these children at three or four years of age; this point is illustrated by a recent study by Barbara Tizard of children raised in residential nurseries.[7] She followed the progress of four groups of children for their first four years. One group spent the first four years in residential nurseries; one group spent two years in nurseries and were then adopted by middle-class families; one group spent two years in residential nurseries and were then restored to their own mothers. Finally, a group of family-reared children were observed as a comparison.

The results are most important for our ideas on the subject of this book. The children who spent their first two years in the nursery had never had the constant individual loving care of one person, attentive in providing comfort when they were distressed. By two years old, they were rather different in their social responses from the children brought up in families. While they did have preferences among the institution staff, they behaved toward them more like one-year-olds than two-year-olds. They ran to be picked up if a familiar nurse came in and cried if she left the room. In their language development they were behind, although their nonverbal intelligence was average. However, at four years of age all the children adopted into middle-class families had developed very good relationships with their new parents; the experience of the first two years had not impaired their ability to become attached. What is more, their language and intellectual development was also very good, better than that of the working-class children who had lived all their lives in their own families. Again, the experience of the first two years had not left an indelible mark on their intellectual ability. Interestingly, the language and intellectual ability of the children who had remained in the nursery for the full four years also greatly improved. Although they had been slow at two, they were now no longer backward in the language, and indeed their language development was considerably ahead of that of the group of children who had been restored to their own mothers. (Most of these mothers were living in hard circumstances, often unsupported and with many children.)

These results do present a challenge to the idea that sensitive individual care and comfort are essential for normal development. But there are several things we should be cautious about. First, in spite of the fact that there were no differences in language development as assessed on an IQ test, there may well have been differences in the way the groups used language in their everyday life which a test would not reveal. We just do not know what sort of difference varying early experiences will make in the children's use of language and what difference, if any, the variation in their use of language will make in their later intellectual development. Courtney Cazden has pointed out that the differences in language between social classes exist primarily in the way language is used in everday life, rather than in the basic linguistic skills.[8]

A second point of caution is that differences in the social behavior and relationships between nursery-reared children and those brought up in families may appear later. And third, the differences in the social behavior of the children brought up in nurseries may in themselves make a great difference in their later intellectual achievement. By four years the children reared in institutions showed a variety of patterns of attachment behavior. Many were clinging and markedly attention-seeking. The nurses also complained of their shallow affections: most of them seemed "not to care deeply about anyone." Some, indeed, seemed emotionally detached from adults.

Nevertheless, the study should make us aware that we may have underestimated the adaptability of the developing child. In summary, two points require particular stress. First, children who are deprived of the experience of individualized comfort and attention in the first two years of life are not incapable of forming deep and lasting attachments when the opportunity is given to them later. Second, we do not really have grounds for supposing that differences in mothers' responses to distress in the first year will affect the children's intellectual ability as they get older, although differences in attentive interest in their babies do appear to affect development while they are still under eighteen months.

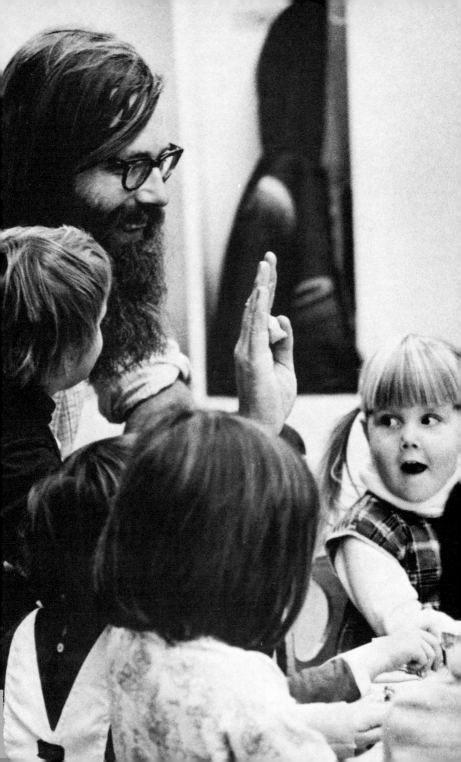

10 / So What?

Our discussion of distress and comfort in the early months has focused on the parent's response to distress as one aspect of a larger question: How does the early relationship between a child and those who care for him affect his later development? We know what a complicated issue this is, but at least we are now beginning to understand the most useful questions to ask about it. Three particular centers of interest seem especially exciting.

One is a change in our interest in "mothering"—a new awareness that attachment grows through reciprocal interaction rather than through the relief of needs like hunger, that what happens in the comfortable play and exchange between mother and baby may be of crucial importance. We are also beginning to grasp how dangerous it may be to have too simple a notion of maternal sensitivity.

A second new interest is our increased appreciation of the importance of the child's contribution to these interactions. We can only understand the growth of the child's relationship with his parents if we see them as interacting *pairs* from the earliest days, and we can only understand the origin of later individual differences between children if we take real account of differences from birth.

The third special point is the new focus on the potential importance of the earliest exchanges between mother and baby for the baby's developing powers of understanding—a new approach to the relation between the baby's emotional development and his intellectual development.

These theoretical ideas are still not very closely articulated in relation to the enormously complicated and detailed pattern of human development. They are closer to stabs in the dark than they are to maps of a fully discovered country. But can we provide any firm practical guidance for the real-life decisions that people looking after children have to face? Let us look briefly at some of the practical implications of this discussion of distress and comfort.

First it is clear that there are great individual differences between babies in how tense and fretful they are and in how difficult it is to pacify them in the early weeks. Parents should not be made to feel responsible for these problems, or for regular evening crying or night waking. The central question of whether a mother who responds quickly to crying is or is not encouraging the crying and dependency must remain open. We do know that other aspects of the mother's social responsiveness, her talking, her enjoyment of and response to her baby's talking, play an important part in encouraging his lively participation in interaction and his intellectual development during the first eighteen months or so. But the recent emphasis on "good" mothering and "appropriate" mothering is not always helpful; it readily promotes blame and guilt for mothers whose babies cry a lot, and a lack of sympathy for those who find continual crying overpowering.

The best pattern of caregiving for a mother and a baby will have to be one that takes account of the needs of both. Dogmatic general advice cannot take much account of individual differences. It is often easier to be clear about what you yourself can stand as a parent than it is to be clear about what the consequences of a particular course of caregiving would be. Finally, there are some clear practical findings.

Mothers who are breastfeeding may expect frequent fussing and wakefulness in the early weeks. If they can manage to feed frequently in response to this fussing, they have a greater chance of success in breastfeeding.

The relationships that have been uncovered between the course of labor and delivery and differences between babies should alert us to the danger of elaborate interventions in birth procedures. Difficult labors, heavy maternal medication, separation of babies in special-care units—all make the early interaction between mother and child more difficult.

We are now beginning to understand in more detail why such age-old soothing techniques as swaddling, rocking, and suckling are effective in calming babies, but it is notable that these care-giving techniques are rarely discussed with young mothers of first babies, who have to discover them for themselves.

Many mothers feel anxious about leaving their babies with other people. But we have learned that it is a definite advantage for the child to get accustomed to being looked after occasion-ally by someone other than his mother: he will then be less ex-posed to distress if he *has* to be left. John Bowlby himself, so often misinterpreted on this issue, has said that it is an excellent plan to have babies and small children cared for now and then by someone else. This point is underlined by what we know about the long-term effects of hospital admissions—children who are very dependent on their mothers or unused to separa-tion are found to be more vulnerable.

Further, if the substitute mothering care is continuous and consistent rather than frequently changing, and if it is warm and friendly, there is no evidence that a child's emotional develop-ment will be adversely affected by daily separations from his mother. Group day-care situations, when well organized, have been shown to have no immediate adverse effects on the devel-opment of children. The fact that so many mothers today have to leave their young children in order to work lends urgency to our search for exactly what substitute mothering is adequate for the child's happiness and comfort. At present there is no good reason to believe that the children of working mothers suffer in later life.

In these ways what we have already learned of the role of dis-tress and comfort in the child's development can tell us some-thing about how we should act as parents. It is of course very much less than it would be nice or reassuring for parents to know. As parents we have to hope that we know what we are doing with our children: to trust our eyes and our feelings. As scientists we have to recognize how little we can yet *know* any-thing of the sort, and we have a duty not to pretend to know any more than we do in fact know. Scientific modesty is not a virtue, it is an obligation. And when what we are speaking of is what from the beginning makes for human joy and human pain, this is an obligation we should take seriously.

References
Suggested Reading
Index

References

2 The Newborn Baby

1. O. Wasz-Hoeckert, J. Lind, V. Vuorenkoski, T. Partanen, and E. Valanné, *The Infant Cry* (London: Heinemann Medical Books, 1968; Philadelphia: Lippincott, 1968).
2. P.H. Wolff, "The Natural History of Crying and Other Vocalisations in Infancy." In B.M. Foss, ed., *Determinants of Infant Behaviour IV* (London: Methuen, 1969).
3. J.F. Bernal, "Crying During the First Ten Days, and Maternal Responses, *Developmental Medicine and Child Neurology*, 1972, *14*, 362-372.
4. L.W. Sander, G. Stechter, P. Burns, and H. Julia, "Early Mother-Infant Interaction and Twenty-Four-Hour Patterns of Activity and Sleep," *Journal of the American Academy of Child Psychiatry*, 1970, *9*, 103-123.
5. T.B. Brazelton, *Neonatal Assessment Scale* (London: Heinemann Medical Books, 1973).
6. F.D. Horowitz, P.A. Self, L.Y. Paden, R. Culp, K. Laub, E. Boyd, and M.E. Mann, "Newborn Test and Four-Week Retest on a Normative Population Using the Brazelton Newborn Assessment Procedure." Paper presented to the Society for Research in Child Development, Minneapolis, 1971.
7. H.A. Moss, "Sex, Age and State as Determinants of Mother-Infant Interaction," *Merrill-Palmer Quarterly*, 1967, *13*, 19-37.
8. D.G. Freedman and N. Freedman, "Behavioural Differences Between Chinese-American and European-American Newborns," *Nature*, 1969, *224*, 1227.
9. T.B. Brazelton and G.A. Collier, "Infant Development in the Zincanteco Indians of Southern Mexico," *Paediatrics*, 1969, *44*, 274-290.
10. Horowitz et al., "Newborn Test."

3 Why Is the Baby Crying?

1. P.H. Wolff, *The Causes, Controls, and Organisation of Behaviour in the Neonate* (New York: International Universities Press, 1966).
2. S.J. Hutt, H.G. Lenard, and H.F.R. Prechtl, "Psychophysiological Studies in Newborn Infants," *Advances in Child Behavior 4* (New York: Academic Press, 1969).

3. P.H. Wolff, "The Natural History of Crying and Other Vocalisations in Early Infancy." In B.M. Foss, ed., *Determinants of Infant Behaviour IV* (London: Methuen, 1969).

4. R.S. Illingworth, "Three Months Colic," *Archives of Disease in Childhood*, 1954, *29*, 165-174.

5. A.J. Ambrose, Discussion contribution in J.A. Ambrose, ed., *Stimulation in Early Infancy* (New York: Academic Press, 1969).

6. Y. Brackbill, "Cumulative Effects of Continuous Stimulation on Arousal Level in Infants," *Child Development*, 1971, *42*, 17-26.

7. L.S. Benjamin, "The Beginnings of Thumb-Sucking," *Child Development*, 1967, *38*, 1965-1968.

4 Changes over the Early Months

1. L.J. Yarrow, "The Development of Focused Relationships During Infancy." In H.J. Hellmuth, *Exceptional Infant*, vol. 1 (New York: Brunner-Mazel, 1967).

2. G.W. Bronson, "Infants' Reactions to Unfamiliar Persons and Novel Objects," *Monographs of the Society for Research in Child Development*, 1972, *148*, 37.

3. D.O. Hebb, "On the Nature of Fear," *Psychological Review*, 1946, *53*, 259-276.

4. L.A. Sroufe, E. Waters, and L. Matas, "Contextual Determinants of Infant Affective Response." In M. Lewis and L.A. Rosenblum, eds., *The Origins of Fear* (New York: Wiley, 1974).

5. J. Kagan, "Discrepancy, Temperament, and Infant Distress." In Lewis and Rosenblum, *The Origins of Fear.*

6. M. Lewis, and J. Brooks, "Self, Other and Fear: Infants' Reactions to People." In Lewis and Rosenblum, *The Origins of Fear.*

7. H.L. Rheingold and C.O. Eckerman, "Fear of the Stranger: A Critical Examination." In H.W. Reese, ed., *Advances of Child Development and Behaviour* (New York: Academic Press, in press).

8. I. Bretherton and M.D.S. Ainsworth, "Response of One-Year-Olds to a Stranger in a Strange Situation." In Lewis and Rosenblum, *The Origins of Fear.*

9. M. Lewis, "The Meaning of a Response, or Why Researchers in Infant Behaviour Should Be Oriental Metaphysicians," *Merrill-Palmer Quarterly*, 1967, *13*, 7-18.

10. Kagan, "Discrepancy, Temperament, and Infant Distress."

11. J. Piaget, *The Origins of Intelligence in Children* (New York: Norton Library, 1963).

12. E. Bates, L. Camaioni, and I. Volterra, "The Acquisition of Per-

formatives prior to Speech," *Merrill-Palmer Quarterly*, 1975, *21*, no. 3, 205-226.

5 Child and Parent in the Early Months

1. E.H. Erikson, "Growth and Crises of the Healthy Personality." In M.J.E. Senn, ed., *Symposium on the Healthy Personality* (New York: Macy Foundation, 1950).
2. S. Freud, "Inhibitions, Symptoms and Anxiety." In *Standard Edition of Complete Psychological Works of Sigmund Freud*, vol. 20 (London: Hogarth Press, 1926), p. 167.
3. R.M. Walters and R.D. Palke, "Social Motivation, Dependency and Susceptibility to Social Influence." In L. Berkovitz, ed., *Advances in Experimental Social Psychology*, vol. 1 (New York: Academic Press, 1964).
4. L.W. Sander, "Comments on Regulation and Organization in the Early Infant-Caretaker System." In R.J. Robinson, ed., *Brain and Early Behavior* (New York: Academic Press, 1969).
5. J. Bowlby, *Attachment and Loss, I: Attachment* (London: Hogarth Press, 1969; New York: Basic Books, 1969).
6. M.D.S. Ainsworth and S.M. Bell, "Attachment, Exploration and Separation: Illustrated by the Behaviour of One-Year-Olds in a Strange Situation," *Child Development*, 1970, *41*, 49-67.
7. I.C. Kaufman, "Mother-Infant Relations in Monkeys and Humans: A Reply to Professor Hinde." In N.F. White, ed., *Ethology and Psychiatry* (Ontario: University of Toronto Press, 1973).
8. F. Rebelsky and R. Black, "Crying in Infancy," *Journal of Genetic Psychology*, 1972, *121*, 49-57.
9. S.M. Bell and M.D.S. Ainsworth, "Infant Crying and Maternal Responsiveness," *Child Development*, 1972, *43*, 1171-1190.
10. A.K. Clarke-Stewart, "Interactions Between Mothers and Their Young Children: Characteristics and Consequences," *Monographs of the Society for Research in Child Development*, 1973, *153*.

6 Crying, Comfort, and Attachments

1. H.R. Schaffer and P.E. Emerson, "The Development of Social Attachments in Infancy," *Monographs of the Society for Research in Child Development*, 1964, *29*, 94.
2. M. Rutter, *Maternal Deprivation Reassessed* (Harmondsworth and New York: Penguin, 1972).
3. S.K. Escalona and H.H. Corman, "The Impact of the Mother's

Presence upon Behaviour: The First Year," *Human Development*, 1971, *14*, 2-15.

4. M.D.S. Ainsworth and B.A. Wittig, "Attachment and Exploratory Behaviour of One-Year-Olds in a Strange Situation." In B.M. Foss, ed., *Determinants of Infant Behaviour IV* (London: Methuen, 1969).

5. Schaffer and Emerson, "The Development of Social Attachments in Infancy."

6. D.J. Stayton and M.D.S. Ainsworth, "Individual Differences in Infant Responses to Brief Everyday Separations as Related to Other Infant and Maternal Behaviors." *Developmental Psychology*, 1973, *9*, 226-235.

7 The Response to Longer Separations

1. J. Bowlby, *Attachment and Loss, II: Separation: Anxiety and Anger* (London: Hogarth Press, 1973, p. 8; New York: Basic Books, 1973).

2. M. Stacey, R. Dearden, R. Pill, and D. Robinson, *Hospitals, Children and Their Families: The Report of a Pilot Study* (London: Routledge, 1970).

3. D.T.A. Vernon, J.M. Foley, R.R. Sipowicz, and J.L. Schulman, *The Psychological Responses of Children to Hospitalization and Illness* (Springfield, Ill.: C.C. Thomas, 1965).

4. C.M. Heinicke and I.J. Westheimer, *Brief Separations* (London: Longmans, 1965; New York: International Universities Press, 1966).

5. M. Rutter, "Parent-Child Separation: Psychological Effects on the Children," *Journal of Child Psychology and Psychiatry*, 1971, *12*, 233-260.

6. J.W.B. Douglas, "Early Hospital Admissions and Later Disturbance of Behaviour and Learning," *Developmental Medicine and Child Neurology*, 1975, *17*, 456-480.

7. J. and J. Robertson, "Young Children in Brief Separation, I, II, and III," *Tavistock Child Development Research Unit*, 1967, 1968a, 1968b.

8. L. Kohlberg, "Stage and Sequence: The Cognitive Developmental Approach to Socialization." In D.A. Goslin, ed., *Handbook of Socialization: Theory and Research* (Chicago: Rand McNally, 1969).

9. E. Maccoby and J.C. Masters, "Attachment and Dependency." In P.H. Mussen, ed., *Carmichael's Manual of Child Psychology*, vol. 2 (New York: Wiley, 1970).

8 Other Cultures

1. I. DeVore and M.J. Konner, "Infancy in Hunter-Gatherer Life: An Ethological Perspective." In White, *Ethology and Psychiatry*. See also I. DeVore and R.B. Lee, eds., *Kalahari Hunter-Gatherers* (Cambridge: Harvard University Press, 1976).
2. M. Mead, *Sex and Temperament in Three Primitive Societies* (London: Routledge and Kegan Paul, 1935; New York: Dell paperback).
3. W. Caudill and H. Weinstein, "Maternal Care and Infant Behavior in Japan and America," *Psychiatry*, 1969, *32*, 12-43.
4. C. Du Bois, *The People of Alor* (Cambridge: Harvard University Press, 1960).

9 The Development of Understanding

1. A.F. Korner and R. Grobstein, "Visual Alertness as Related to Soothing in Neonates," *Child Development*, 1966, *37*, 867-876.
2. S.K. Escalona, *The Roots of Individuality* (New York: Aldine, 1968).
3. D. Wood, J.S. Bruner, and G. Ross, "The Role of Tutoring in Problem Solving," *Journal of Child Psychology and Psychiatry*, 1976, in press.
4. L.J. Yarrow, J.L. Rubenstein, F.A. Pederson, and J.M. Jankowski, "Dimensions of Early Stimulation and Their Differential Effects on Infant Development," *Merrill-Palmer Quarterly*, 1972, *18*, no. 3, 205-218.
5. Clarke-Stewart, "Interactions Between Mothers and Their Young Children."
6. S.M. Bell, "The Development of the Concept of the Object as Related to Infant-Mother Attachment," *Child Development*, 1970, *41*, 291-311.
7. J.F. Dunn, "Patterns of Early Interaction: Continuities and Consequences." In H.R. Schaffer, ed., *Interactions in Infancy: The Loch Lomond Symposium* (London and New York: Academic Press, 1977, in press).
8. B. Tizard and J. Rees, "The Effects of Early Institutional Rearing on the Behaviour Problems and Affectional Relationships of Four-Year-Old Children," *Journal of Child Psychology and Psychiatry*, 1975, *16*, 61-73.
9. C.M. Cazden, "The Situation: A Neglected Source of Social Class Differences in Language Use," *Journal of Social Issues*, 1970, *26*, no. 2, 35-60.

Suggested Reading

John Bowlby, *Attachment and Loss, I: Attachment* (London: Hogarth Press, 1968; New York: Basic Books, 1969) and *Attachment and Loss, II: Anxiety and Anger* (London: Hogarth Press, 1973; New York: Basic Books, 1973). In these important books, Bowlby develops his ideas on the child's relationship with its mother, based on years of experience in clinical and research work. These books have had a profound influence on attitudes toward and ideas about mothering, and about the care of children in residential institutions and hospitals, and they have generated a new approach to the study of early social development.

Charles Darwin, *The Expression of Emotions in Man and Animal* (London: Murray, 1872; Chicago and London: University of Chicago Press, 1965). A classic study of the relation between behavior and feeling in both language-using animals and animals without language.

John and Elizabeth Newson, *Infant Care in an Urban Community* (Chicago: Aldine, 1963; Harmondsworth: Penguin, 1965). A fascinating study of baby care in Nottingham, based on interviews with 700 families. What parents actually do, and how they feel about and react to the pleasures and difficulties of looking after a young baby, are vividly presented in the parents' own words.

Michael Rutter, *Maternal Deprivation Reassessed* (Harmondsworth and New York: Penguin, 1972). Rutter reconsiders the issue of the effects of separation and "deprivation" in a brilliantly succinct and clear review of the research, focusing on why and how children are affected by different experiences, and raising further questions about the nature of the relationship between mother and child.

Peter Wolff, "The Natural History of Crying," in B. M. Foss, ed., *Determinants of Infant Behaviour*, IV (London: Methuen, 1969). An illuminating account of detailed observations of eighteen babies over the first month of life. The different causes and sounds of crying, effects on the parent, and the consequences of different types of parental response are all explored.

Index

Adolescence, problems in related to early separations, 77

Age differences: in causes of distress, 2; in reactions to people, 29-30, 36-37; in reactions to strange situations, 31-35; in separation protest, 68, 74

Ainsworth, Mary Salter, 38, 54, 102; on crying and attention, 58; on crying at mother's absence, 64; on attachment bond, 65; on security of attachment, 66; on separation protest, 69

Alertness, and intellectual development, 96-97

Alor, people of, 90-91

Ambrose, Anthony, 23

Animals, fear of discrepancy in, 31. *See also* Apes; Monkeys

Anxiety of mother, and crying by infant, 12-13

Apes, and attachment theory, 53. *See also* Chimpanzees

Arapesh (New Guinea), 88

Arousal, levels of, 18

Attachment: differences in, 63-65; forms of, 65-70; origin of differences in, 68-70; of !Kong children, 92

Attachment theory, 53-57; role of crying in, 55-56; and differences between babies, 58. *See also* Bowlby, John

Attention: -getting, 2; -seeking, 82

Bates, Elisabeth, 43

Bell, Sylvia, 54; on crying and attention, 58; on mother's departure, 64; on mother's responsive-ness, and object permanence, 101-102

Benedek, Therese, 49

Benjamin, Lorna, 24-25

Biological adaptation, and social behavior, 92-93

Birth cry, 5

Bowlby, John, 49; attachment theory, 53-57, 79, 92; on response to separation, 73, 77; on special relationship to mother, 78, 81; on occasional separations, 111

Brackbill, Yvonne, 23-24

Brazelton, T. Berry, 11, 14

Breastfeeding: and infant crying, 8, 27-28, 110; composition of milk, 93

Bretherton, Inge, 38

Bronson, Gordon, 30, 32; on negative reactions to strangers, 36-37, 40

Brooks, Jeanne, 34

Bruner, Jerome, 23; on play periods and development of skills, 99-100

Cambridge study, 8-9; on amount of crying, 11; on medication of mother, 12, 13; on hunger, 20; on evening crying, 22; on interrupted feeding, 27; on attention to crying, 59; on later intelligence, 103-104

Campos, John, 37

Carpenter, Genevieve, 31

Caudill, William, 89-90

Causes of crying: changes in, 2; states of consciousness, 17-20; hunger, 20; temperature, 20-21; clothing and contact, 21; pain and evening crying, 21-22; sudden stimulation, 22; changes in during early months, 27-29

Cazden, Courtney, 106

Child, the, importance of contribution to relationships by, 109

Child-parent relationship: psychoanalytical approach to, 47-50; social-learning approach to, 50-53, 58; attachment theory approach to, 53-57, 58; differences between babies, 57-60; new directions in, 60-61

Chimpanzees: play and social behavior in, 82; frustration and learning in, 97; play and skills in, 99-100

Chinese babies, crying of, 14

Circumcision, 13-14

Clarke-Stewart, Alison, 59-60, 101

Class differences, in interpretation of cries, 9

Colic, and evening crying, 21-22

Comfort: sources of, 22-25; changes in during early months, 27-29; objects of, 38-39

Communication, in relationship with mother, 60, 95, 96-97

Confidence, development of, 48-49. *See also* Security

Consciousness, states of, 17-20. *See also* Intentional crying

Contact: as a comfort, 21, 53; physical vs. social, 84; and states of alertness, 96

Corman, Helen, 66

Cries: kinds of, 5-6; identified by parents, 6, 7-9

Cross-cultural studies: of newborns' irritability, 14; of childrearing, 87-93; cautions related to, 92-93

Crying patterns, and child's development, 2

Cultural differences: in source of security, 82-83; complexity of, 87-89; in social behavior, 92-93

Darwin, Charles, 55

Day care, 83-84, 111

Differentiation, of child from others, 48

Discrepancy hypothesis, 31; difficulties with, 32-35

Distress: changing causes of, 2; and ideas of development, 3; causes of, 20-22; at separation, 78-80

Douglas, James, 76-77

DuBois, Cora, 90-91

Dunn, Judy, 8

Early care, and amount of crying, 11

Early months, changes in: crying and comforting, 27-29; reactions to people, 29-30; reactions to strangers, 30-35; nature of wariness, 35-39; individual differences, 39-41; crying intentionally, 41-44

Eckerman, Carol, 37

Emerson, Peggy, 63, 68

Erikson, Erik, 49

Escalona, Sibylle, 49, 66, 98-99

Evening crying, 21-22, 110

Exploration, and security, 65-67

Father: attachment to, 64; separation from, 78, 83

Feeding, demand vs. schedule, 8

Freedman, D.G. and N., 14

Freud, Anna, 48, 49

Freud, Sigmund, 47, 48; on gratification, 49-50; on frustration and learning, 97

Frustration and teasing, 27, 28-29; and learning, 97

Grobstein, Rose, 96-97

Harlow, Harry, 54; on security and exploration, 67, 81
Hebb, Donald, 31
Heinicke, Christoph, 73, 76, 78
Hinde, Robert, 54, 75
Horowitz, Frances, 12
Hospital, 111; separation caused by admission to, 74-77; distress caused by, 78-80; effects of stay in, 99
Hunger cry, 5
Hunter-gatherer societies, 91-93
Hutt, John, 18

Illingworth, Ronald, 21-22
Individual differences: in newborns' irritability, 9-14, 110; persistence of, 39-41; in child-parent relationship, 109
Intellectual development. See Understanding
Intentional crying, and intentional behavior, 41-44

Japanese, childrearing by, 89-90

Kagan, Jerome, 33, 40
Kaufman, Charles, 55
Kibbutzim, studies of children in, 64, 83
Kohlberg, Lawrence, 81
Korner, Anneliese, 96-97
!Kung, 87, 91, 92-93

Labor and delivery: and individual differences in infants, 10, 11-13; sex differences in reaction to, 13; difficulties in, 110
Language: linked to mother-child understanding, 61, 95; setting for learning, 100; ability in, and early care, 105; everyday use of, 106
Lewis, Michael, 34, 35, 40
Lind, John, 5

Maccoby, Eleanor, 82
Masters, John, 82
Mead, Margaret, 88-89
Means and ends, dissociation of, 42
Medication of mother, and individual differences in infants, 11-13
Monkeys: thumbsucking in, 25; importance of contact with mothers, 53, 54-55; security and exploration, 67, 81; reactions to separation from mothers, 75, 76, 77; basis of social interaction among, 81
Moss, Howard, 13
Mothering styles: and future development of child, 102-106; as reciprocal interaction, 109
Mothers: infants' ability to discriminate, 29-30; permanence of, 44; psychoanalysis on mother-child relationship, 47-50; effect of differences between, 51-53; importance of contact with, 53-55; protection as function of, 54; distress at separation from, 68-70; effect of longer separations from, 75-76; relationships with, and intellectual development, 99-101
Mundugumor, 88-89

Newborn, study of crying by, 5

Object permanence, 101

Pain cry, 5
Parenting, styles of, 41. See also Mothering styles
Parents, cries identified by, 6, 7-9
Parke, R.D., 51
People: infants' interest in, 28; changes in reaction to, 29-30
Physical situation, as cause of distress, 2
Piaget, Jean: on power of recall, 30;

on dissociating means and ends, 42-44; on tension, 98; on object permanence, 101

Play: and development of social behavior, 81; and development of skills, 99

Plooij, Franz, 97

Prechtl, Heinz, 18

Psychoanalysis, and child-parent relationship, 47-50

Psychological situation, as cause of distress, 2

Rebelsky, Freda, 57

Recall, powers of, 30

Relationships: distress as key to, 2-3; importance of differences in, 63; security and development of, 80-83; with other children, 83

Rheingold, Harriet, 37

Richards, Martin, 8

Robertson, James, 77, 79

Robertson, Joyce, 79

Rocking, 23, 110

Ross, Gail, 99

Rutter, Michael, 65; on longer separations, 76, 77, 78

Sander, Louis, 11; on crying behavior and infant care, 51-52, 56

Schaffer, Rudolph, 63, 64, 68, 99

Security: from contact, 21, 53; of attachment, 65-67; and separation, 67-70; physical vs. psychological, 84; prerequisite to learning, 100

Self, infant's concept of, 34-35, 48

Self-quieting: infant ability in, 20; by sucking, 23

Separation protest, 67; differences in, 68-70

Separations, longer, 73-85, 111; degrees of distress, 74-77; previous, 74-75; causes of distress, 78-80; amelioration of distress, 79-80; and social behavior, 80-83; day care, 83-84; physical contact and security, 84-85

Sex differences: in irritability, 13-14; in distress at separation, 74; in physical contact for security, 84

Sharing and communication, basic to development of social behavior, 81

Siblings: order of, and mother's reaction to crying, 9; comfort from, 78; and social behavior, 81

Sleep, stages of, 17-19

Social behavior: relation of security to development of, 80-83; related to early care, 106

Social-learning theory, 50-53; effect of differences between mothers, 51-53; and differences between babies, 58

Spectograms: of infant cries, 6; in diagnosis of abnormality, 6-7

Spitz, René, 49, 50, 97

Spoiling, attitudes toward, and response to crying, 9, 59, 87

Sroufe, Alan, 33-34; use of heartrate by, 36, 37

Stacey, M., 74

Stimulation: constant, as comfort, 23-24; of comfort objects, 39

Strangers: changing reactions to, 30-35; discrepancy hypothesis, 32-35; children as, 34; negative reactions to, 36

Sucking, comfort from, 23, 110; thumbsucking, 24-25

Swaddling, 21, 23, 24, 110

Temperament, and reaction to separation, 74

Thumbsucking, 24-25

Tizard, Barbara, 104
Trevarthen, Colwyn, 96-97

Understanding, development of: and response to absence of familiar people, 29-30; and differences in wariness, 41; and intentional behavior, 42-44; state of baby related to, 95-98; and interaction with adults, 98-102, 109; and mothering styles, 102-106
Uraguayan babies, 14

Vernon, D.T.A., 75

Walters, R.M., 51
Wariness, nature of, 35-39; heart-rate as measure of, 36; changes in nature of, 36-37; complications in, 38
Wasz-Hoeckert, Olé, 5
Weinstein, Helen, 89-90
Westheimer, Ilse, 73, 76, 78
Wittig, Barbara, 66
Wolff, Peter, 6, 23; study of crying by, 18-20, 95-96; on hunger, 20; on temperature, 20-21; on clothing and contact, 21; on teasing, 27, 29; on recognition of mother, 29
Wood, David, 99

Yarrow, Leon, 29, 100-101

Zinacanteco Indians, 14